THE BACK AND BEYOND

Dr Paul Sherwood, consultant in physical medicine, trained at Cambridge University and the Westminster Hospital. After achieving a degree in medicine he worked as a house surgeon at Westminster Hospital, and later at Barts before becoming a consultant at a number of hospitals.

Dr Sherwood set up his own private clinic in London where he has been developing his own form of physical medicine over a period of 40 years.

Following the success of the original publication of *The Back and Beyond*, Dr Sherwood received many enquiries from readers about the effects of back problems on their sex lives. He has added a new chapter on 'Your Back and Sex' for this new edition of his acclaimed book.

THE BACK
AND BEYOND

The hidden effects of back
problems on your health

Revised Edition

Dr Paul Sherwood

ARROW

Dedicated to my Father who passed on to me some of his brains and a great deal of the knowledge that started the subject of this book

First published by Arrow Books, 1992

3 5 7 9 10 8 6 4 2

Arrow Books Limited
Random House, 20 Vauxhall Bridge Road, London SW1V 2SA

Random House Australia (Pty) Limited
20 Alfred Street, Milsons Point, Sydney,
New South Wales 2061, Australia

Random House New Zealand Limited
18 Poland Road, Glenfield
Auckland 10, New Zealand

Random House South Africa (Pty) Limited
PO Box 337, Bergvlei, South Africa

Random House UK Limited Reg. No. 954009

ISBN 0 09 943841 0

Printed and bound in Great Britain by
Cox & Wyman Ltd, Reading, Berkshire

CONTENTS

AUTHOR'S NOTE

This book is concerned with *non-specific* back pain. It is important that all back problems be given a proper medical assessment to eliminate all diagnosable causes for it is only after full investigation that a verdict of non-specific back pain can be reached.

I would also like to stress that my recommended treatment is always given alongside, not instead of, other medical care. All back sufferers should seek medical advice and help, especially for the complications that can occur with back trouble.

The various secondary effects of back trouble, such as peptic ulcer or arthritic joint, should also be medically supervised. These conditions may give rise to serious complications and it is important that you continue to be supervised by your own doctor or specialist during treatment to the back. The secondary illness will usually clear up within a few weeks of treatment to the back and the nerve centre, but it makes sense to attack the problem on all fronts, especially if the local symptoms are bad.

ACKNOWLEDGEMENTS

To Mary Atkinson, for recasting this book so that academic stodge became readable English. Mr Toby Judge, for the hours of expert professional guidance without which this book could have been published a year earlier. Mr Alexander Patt, without whose persistence in high quarters this book would never have seen the light of day.

My family, staff and patients, who put up with me for the three years and gave much help and guidance over this period.

INTRODUCTION

'But doctor, I only leaned forward to look in the mirror. I wanted to see if I had a pimple on my chin. The next thing I knew my back became agonizingly painful and I haven't been able to move for three days.'

'I am hoping you can do something. For the last six years I've had acute attacks of back pain and have been off work for three or four days each time.'

'If I do anything – carrying the shopping, a little work in the garden, or, worst of all, lifting up my three-year-old daughter – I get bad pain in my back within twenty-four hours. It is spoiling my life.'

These are common complaints from patients coming to me for consultation. Most say their GPs could not help. Some back-pain sufferers are told that the pain is psychosomatic, or all in the mind, others that they should expect back trouble with their advancing years or that they must simply learn to live with it.

Most back sufferers find their own temporary solutions, just as you probably have your own 'secret' for coping with the pain. Unhappy with the treatment offered by doctors, some people find their own form of pain relief such as swimming, yoga or self-manipulation. Many try a variety of treatments including acupuncture, osteopathy, relaxation techniques, chiropractic and faith healing. These practitioners often offer immediate pain relief where doctors have provided little help. But most patients find that their back problems still recur . . .

'I go to an osteopath or chiropractor each time I have an attack of pain but he doesn't seem to be able to stop my back from "going out" again. What I want is permanent relief.'

'I have been going to an osteopath for twelve years for each attack of pain and have always been satisfied. But on this last occasion he could not help. What else can I do?'

People who suffer from 'non-specific' back pain have to live with aches that may restrict their activities; they also live with the fear of a possible severe attack of pain. On the whole, sufferers have little positive help from the medical profession. When someone has a heart attack he would usually go straight to a heart specialist, confident in the knowledge that he would receive the best care and expertise for his condition. Is it not strange that back trouble takes people more often to the large army of alternative practitioners and not to the medical consultants? So the question that we must ask is why do back sufferers have such little faith in the medical profession? The answer is clear. Osteopaths, chiropractors and others are able to help rapidly and painlessly patients previously confined to bed, to wearing corsets and collars, or undergoing surgery. Indeed, it is doubtful if the treatment of acute pain by osteopaths or chiropractors could be bettered (acute, meaning arising suddenly and of a short duration). It is only in the long-term that these treatments may not prove to be so successful. There is much to be learned from the less orthodox practitioners.

There is some confusion between the treatment itself and the means by which treatment is carried out, such as manipulation, exercises, relaxation, physiotherapy and others. Patients have often told me that they had already had this sort of treatment in the past and that it had helped only temporarily. So they dismissed these manoeuvres as being of little value. What most patients do not realize is that manipulation, ultrasonic waves and 'other treatments' are in fact simply tools to carry out the treatment and are not the treatment itself. It is important to understand this distinction so I would like to expand this point.

Let us suppose a bearing keeps wearing out in a car engine. The repair is to replace the bearing, and spanners and screwdrivers are tools which the garage uses to carry out the repair. If each new bearing also rapidly wears out, then you may well go to another garage for a second opinion. At this garage the mechanic may say that the real problem is that the oil filter is blocked and needs replacing. He will use spanners and screwdrivers to accomplish this. Once the oil filter is renewed the car works perfectly and there is no further trouble.

The mechanic at the second garage used the same tools as at the first but with greater success. By discovering the underlying trouble in the blocked oil filter he could put the tools to more effective use and provide permanent repair.

Ultrasonic waves, massage and manipulation are the equivalent to the spanners and screwdrivers used by the mechanic and similarly they can be used for different purposes with varying degrees of success.

In this book I will show that by treating the basic *cause* of back pain, just as the mechanic at the second garage worked on the underlying problem with the car, it is possible to help back problems to a great extent using techniques and instruments which are widely available.

I will show how and why back trouble needs to be taken a great deal more seriously than most people, including the medical profession, believe. This book puts forward a new theory about the cause of intermittent back pain and for the first time I can offer an explanation as to why – as many alternative practitioners already know – a person with a bad back often suffers from a number of associated complaints, such as tiredness and headaches. These are very often helped by successful treatment to the back.

I will also go one step further and identify many complaints such as ME (Myalgic Encephalomyelitis, or Chronic Fatigue Syndrome), migraine, indigestion and even stomach and duodenal ulcers, and show that they too are caused by back problems. By treating the root cause – in the back – these problems also can usually be cured. We will introduce a so-far-unrecognized disease, which I have named HST. This disease, which is characterized by tiredness, depression, a tensed-up feeling, indigestion, and aches between the shoulders, is making life a misery for many thousands of people. HST is caused by back trouble. With a correct diagnosis it is as easy to treat as the back itself.

In the final chapters there is outlined a treatment which not only can relieve back pain permanently, but also provide long-term help for related illnesses. The treatment, which has proved successful over the past forty years, relies on physical medicine and involves *no risk* to the patient. It is a treatment that could save the health service around two thousand million pounds a year.

My approach to back trouble is holistic, working in the belief that all parts of the body are connected and inter-related. Unlike many of the medical profession, who concentrate on one organ and all the different problems associated with that one part, I concentrate on a *family* of illnesses and whichever part of the body it assails. The orthodox medical principles of my theory are not new but I believe that my reassessment of how they are put together has never been advocated before.

The Back Pain Association (see page 243) estimates that every year over three million Britons consult a family doctor because of back trouble. For well over half these sufferers there is little positive help. They are told that their pain can only be relieved when they suffer a new attack. They are then told that they are cured of their trouble. Until it happens again . . . I do not agree with this principle. I believe that patients with back pain can both be offered immediate relief and be prevented from having recurring bouts if they are given the correct treatment.

This book offers sufferers a more permanent pain relief and provides a better understanding of the fundamental problem. Very many patients are confused because their symptoms do not seem to match the explanation. And treatment so often makes them feel worse. They are puzzled by their pain: Why is it so often worse in the morning? Why do they feel so much better in sunny weather? You will find logical explanations for these and many other seeming paradoxes. You will also find out why, contrary to popular opinion, back pain is not an inevitable part of old age, and poor posture is not to blame for back trouble.

I can offer doctors a new insight into back pain and the serious repercussions that back trouble can have throughout the whole body. Hopefully, it will make doctors give the problem a major rethink and encourage debate among both the medical profession and the general public. As I shall show throughout the book, bed rest has few benefits; surgery is only ever necessary in extreme cases; traction and corsets often make the problem worse and anti-inflammatory drugs all too often have little effect. Alternative practitioners offer more positive help but this is usually only short-term and does little to relieve the underlying problem.

So, you might ask, how is my theory and form of treatment so different? The crux of my theory lies in the fact that the majority of back-pain therapists concentrate on relieving the *present* attack of pain but do little to stop future attacks. I believe that we should be looking beyond the actual attack of pain to the deep-rooted cause. When a patient has intermittent back pain the basic problem is present all the time. The pain is only a result of a change in the underlying problem; by ridding the patient of pain the therapist isn't necessarily doing anything to correct the basic problem.

I believe that all non-specific back pain has its root in an old injury – a fall down stairs, perhaps, or from a hard rugby tackle – which disturbs the spinal column. The back may remain symptomless for many years. Often a minor episode such as leaning over the bar or reaching to pick up a cup may spark off the pain. The pain may come and go over the years but the basic trouble remains, as do the symptoms of the other illnesses already mentioned.

My work over the past forty years has shown that by promoting the recovery of the bruised facet joints, it is possible for a troublesome back to be permanently restored to good health. The 'tools' and techniques of my treatment are widely available in physiotherapy departments all over the country: manipulation, remobilization, massage, ultrasonic waves and surged faradism (which is a controlled electrical current designed to stimulate the muscle). By treating the cause rather than the symptoms, I have given to most of my patients long-lasting relief from both back pain and the associated illnesses.

Already, in Britain, around sixty million working days are lost each year through back pain and the figure is rising. Those days cost the economy around three billion pounds in 1992. On its own the amount is shocking, but think of the days lost through related illnesses. How many millions of pounds are we losing through lack of effective diagnosis and treatment for back pain? In Britain alone, there is a cost of over £350 million to the health service to treat these patients. And that figure is rising. The treatment I suggest can be used as a basis for seeking help through your own doctor or from a suitably trained physiotherapist, osteopath or other therapist in your area.

There are many theories for the cause and relief of back pain, and whilst mine might seem to be just one of the many, my theory has produced an effective treatment which has already relieved thousands and thousands of back pain sufferers. Hopefully this book will help many more people.

Almost everyone who suffers from non-specific back pain can be completely cured with the correct tools and diagnosis. This book will present you with the necessary information to find yours.

1

KNOW YOUR BACK

*The anatomy and function
of your spinal column*

If you are to understand back pain and its related problems it is important that you have some knowledge of how the spine works and the part it plays within the body machine. So, with the help of diagrams, let us consider briefly the anatomy and functions of the spinal column.

The Spinal Column

The spine has three important functions:

- **Support.** As you can see from figure 1.1 on page 18, the spine is an extension of the legs, supporting the whole of the abdomen and thorax (the area between the abdomen and neck) and giving the head a firm base to carry its weight. It acts like a frame, holding apart all the soft tissues and other bones between the legs, the pelvis, the arms, the head and the ribs.
- **Protection.** The spinal column works in association with the ribs to give a measure of protection to the heart and lungs, and, with the pelvis, to protect the lower abdominal organs. Much more importantly, it also encloses the spinal cord. This vital and very vulnerable structure of spinal nerves runs from the brain stem down to the top of the lumbar spine (the

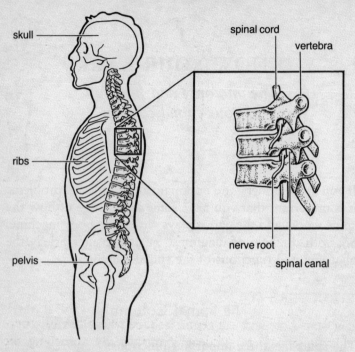

Figure 1.1 The spine is the centre of support, protecting the spinal cord and – with the ribs, skull and pelvis – the organs and nerves in its box. In the inset, note how the spinal cord runs up through the spinal canal in the vertebrae.

part of the spine which runs between the lowest ribs and the hip bones), where it finally divides into the smaller nerves known as the *cauda equina*.

- **Mobility.** The third function is to allow some movement to the trunk, making it possible to either bend backwards and forwards, sideways or to undergo a rotational movement. This means the body can move on the pelvis and the head can move independently from the rest of the trunk. See figure 1.2, on page 19.

18

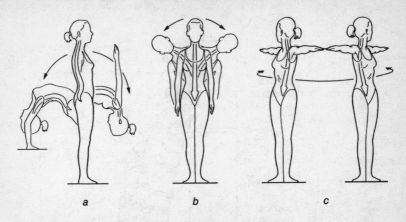

Figure 1.2 For such a strong structure, the spine is enormously flexible, allowing movement: backwards and forwards (*a*), side to side (*b*), and rotationally (*c*).

STRUCTURE

The spinal column is a gentle S-shape whose flexible curve is capable of very sudden alterations. By absorbing the force of unexpected shocks or blows it provides a cushioning effect.

Vertebrae

The spine is made up of twenty-nine small bones called vertebrae, placed one on top of another. Each individual vertebra is shaped rather like a tin of food, round with a flat top and bottom. Most of the vertebrae are separate but five at the bottom are fused into one single bone known as the sacrum. At this point in the spinal column rigidity and strength are more important than flexibility. At the extreme end of the spine is our residual tail called the coccyx, which is made up of a number of jointed bones (see figure 1.3).

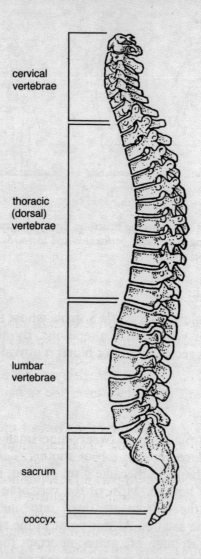

cervical
vertebrae

thoracic
(dorsal)
vertebrae

lumbar
vertebrae

sacrum

coccyx

Figure 1.3 These are the divisions of the spine. It's important to identify which vertebrae are affected before treatment can be undertaken.

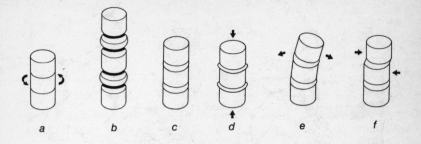

Figure 1.4 The mechanical function of the discs. In diagram *a*, flat surface against flat surface allows only rotational movement; *b* and *c* show these surfaces with an added layer of elastic tissue (the intervertebral discs), permitting all kinds of movement; *d* shows compression, and *e* and *f* illustrate backwards, forwards, side to side, and sliding motions.

Intervertebral discs

The vertebrae are separated from each other by intervertebral discs, which are shaped like old-fashioned pill boxes. Each disc is a sort of fibrous box, which is welded to the vertebrae above and below. The discs are filled with an elastic jelly which gives the spinal column flexibility.

Without these discs the movement of the spine would be very limited. Picture the spinal column as a pile of food tins. Try stacking a few tins top to bottom and you will find that with two hard flat surfaces positioned so near to each other, the only possible movement is rotational. It is impossible for the column to move backwards, forwards, sideways, upwards and downwards without the tins falling off one another. Now try sticking the tins to one another with a half-inch of spongy rubber and there is a full range of movement (see figure 1.4).

Intervertebral discs give the spinal column freedom of

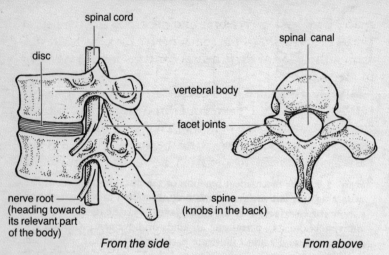

spinal cord

disc

spinal canal

vertebral body

facet joints

nerve root
(heading towards
its relevant part
of the body)

spine
(knobs in the back)

From the side

From above

Figure 1.5 Vertebrae, facet joints, discs and nerves. See how the facet joints form to fit together, providing protection and support.

movement, and provide it with a greater ability to with-stand blows.

Facet joints

With intervertebral discs the structure is flexible, but on its own it is also somewhat floppy. You wouldn't want to entrust your body to such an unstable column. Nature appears to take the same view. It has provided joints known as facet joints to stabilize the back and limit excessive movement. They also make it extremely difficult for vertebrae to become displaced.

Figure 1.5 illustrates how these joints are formed. As you can see, an arch of bone projects from the back of each of the vertebral bodies (vertebrae). Four projections from each arch meet two corresponding ones from the arches above and two from the arches below to form slanting joints called facet joints.

These arches encase and protect the spinal cord. The

spaces between the vertebrae and the arches are the neural canals through which the spinal nerves pass. As figure 1.5 shows, the floor of these neural canals is largely made up of the facet joints.

A nerve associated with each vertebra comes from the enclosed spinal cord, passes out through the canal formed by the arch and facet joint and then goes to the part of the body it supplies. This is the nerve root, which is the base for a nerve in the body. A nerve may form from a number of roots.

As we have already seen, the discs allow a great deal of movement between the vertebrae. It is the discs that enable the vertebrae to squeeze together in a compressional movement, or to turn in a rotational movement. Obviously, it is important to keep this movement to a safe level so Nature provides built-in restrictions in the form of muscles, ligaments, and also the facet joints.

The facet joints bear the brunt of a blow or sharp jolt to the spine. Say, for example, you slip and sit down hard on the floor. The natural curve of the back increases, thus decreasing the effect of the blow. The discs will absorb much of the force by compressing. The facet joints, however, which have restricted movement, may be badly affected. The shock of the jolt could produce more movement than the facet joints are capable of accommodating, and, when given a sharp blow, they may well become damaged.

Similarly, with injuries such as falling flat on your back from a horse, or falling downstairs, the type of jolt sustained in a car accident, or the twisting motion involved in a skiing accident or hard rugby tackle, the facet joints may not be able to cope with the range of attempted movement and are likely to be bruised.

Spinal muscles

Muscles are important to the spinal column, and they have three main functions:

- **Movement.** This is the most obvious function. Many extremely intricate bundles of muscles run up and down the spinal column. These muscles control the movements of the spine – such as bending forward and straightening up, bending from side to side and rotation. They, in turn, are, of course, controlled by the motor centre of the brain. When you decide to perform a function such as walking or picking up an object, the motor centre of the brain is activated and sends a complex series of impulses to the various muscles involved.
- **Maintenance of posture.** Your carriage, when not moving, is sustained by the muscles of the spinal column. When you are sitting or standing you may feel quite relaxed but your muscles are actually working quite hard to maintain the spinal curves and stiffen them so your body stays erect. If your spinal muscles were to be paralysed suddenly, say by the administration of a drug, then your spine would promptly collapse and you would fall in a heap on the floor.

You have little voluntary control over this static posture. It is usually maintained without any conscious effort on your behalf. Sensors determine the positions of the muscles, joints and ligaments and if the posture changes they react by sending impulses to the brain stem and to the cerebellum, or 'little brain', at the base of the brain, which has overall control over your posture. In response, appropriate impulses are then sent out to correct the muscles

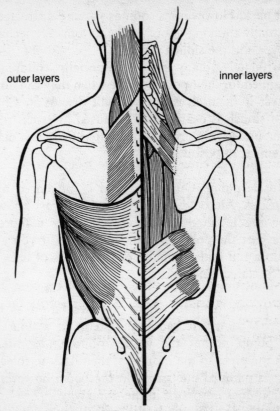

outer layers

inner layers

Figure 1.6 The muscles in the back. Messages are sent to the brain stem and the cerebellum from each layer when any movement occurs, and posture is maintained.

involved and restore the usual posture. Figure 1.6 shows the complex nature of the muscle layers in relation to the spine and the back.

It is a common belief that slouching is slovenly behaviour; however, since posture is controlled by the cerebellum, clearly this is not so. You can momentarily over-ride poor posture by exerting conscious control over the muscles and make an effort to sit or stand with a straight back. However, as soon as you are distracted and stop actually thinking about it, the automatic mechanism takes over and the slouch returns.

Unfortunately, many people, especially children, are reprimanded for their poor posture when they can do little to correct it themselves. As we will discuss in Chapter Three, a slouch is nearly always caused by back trouble. Once the underlying problem is treated there is a marked improvement in posture.

- **Muscle pump.** Our circulation is influenced by the muscles. Although this is one of the least known of the muscle functions, it is crucial that you appreciate the part they play in your circulation if you are to gain a full understanding of the causes of back pain and related illnesses.

Most people tend to regard the circulation as being similar to a domestic radiator system. In a house, the central pump pushes the water round under pressure through the pipes to the radiators, then back to the pump where it is pumped out again. In the body, however, the circulation does not work in the same way.

The heart does resemble the central pump in that it pumps the blood through the pipes – or arteries – to the tissues, but it requires help to pump the blood back along the veins to the heart.

The blood leaves the heart through a large artery called the aorta. It then goes into smaller arteries, which branch off and become even smaller. As their size decreases, the arteries progressively increase the resistance to the flow. The blood eventually passes through the minute arteriols which can expand and contract their diameter considerably, and are responsible for controlling the exact quantity of blood required by the tissues. The blood then flows into

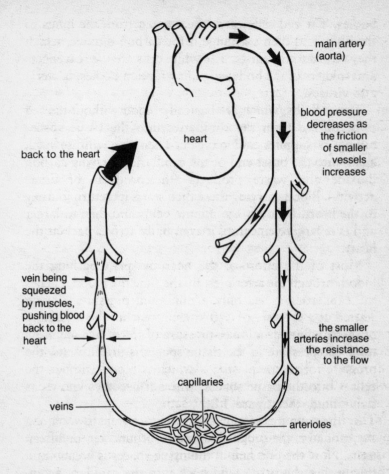

Figure 1.7 The circulation of blood. As blood pressure decreases, the muscles must work to return blood to the heart.

thin-walled vessels called capillaries. See figure 1.7, which illustrates the movement of the blood from the heart, through the body, and back.

Blood is a complex fluid containing both red and white cells, as well as other substances such as salts and antibodies. The red cells carry the oxygen from the lungs to the body and then exchange it for carbon dioxide, which they return to the lungs. The white cells are the scavengers and soldiers of the body, engulfing foreign bodies, bacteria and viruses.

Tissue fluids, which are basically blood without the red cells, diffuse from the capillaries into the tissue spaces taking in supplies and oxygen. Then they diffuse back again into the other end of the capillaries carrying carbon dioxide and waste products (the products of tissue activity). Blood carrying these then starts its return journey to the heart. It flows into minute veins and then to larger and ever larger veins until it eventually arrives back at the heart.

Most of the effort of the heart is spent pushing the blood through the arterioles. By the time the blood reaches the capillaries it has only a minimum pressure. Having started at a pressure of 120 units, it reaches the beginning of the capillary at a lower pressure of thirty-five units. As the basic pressure in the tissue spaces is fifteen units, the pressure forces the plasma – which is blood without the cells – into the tissue spaces, where it becomes known as tissue fluid. (See figure 1.8.)

By the time the blood reaches just over halfway along the capillary, the pressure drops to around ten or fifteen units. Now the pressure in the tissue spaces is greater and this pushes the tissue fluid back into the capillary again. Blood leaves the capillary to go into the veins with a basic pressure of about ten units. This is sufficient – along with the pumping effect of breathing and the constant rhythmic contractions of the vein walls, pushing blood ahead, like a piston – to maintain circulation when you are lying down or sleeping (see figure 1.9). However, as soon as you start to move about, a new pumping force is needed. This is known as the muscle pump.

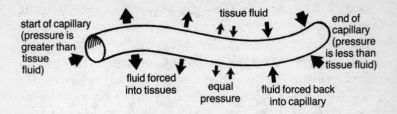

Figure 1.8 The circulation of fluid through a capillary. Higher pressure in the capillaries forces fluid out, and into the tissues. When the tissues reach a higher pressure, fluid is forced back into the capillary. The larger arrows indicate higher pressure.

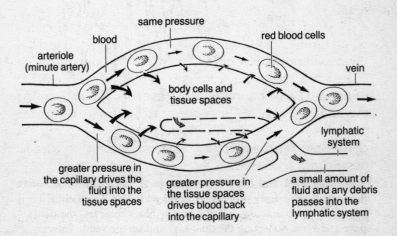

Figure 1.9 A larger view of capillary and tissue circulation.

The muscle pump at work

When a person is active, large volumes of blood need to be returned to the heart, for the greater the level of activity,

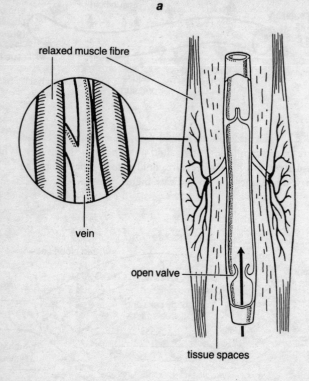

Figure 1.10 The muscle pump. In diagram *a*, the relaxed muscle fibres allow veins and tissue spaces to fill with fluid. Diagram *b* indicates how contracting, bulging muscle fibres compress the tissue space and veins, squeezing the fluid into and up the veins. Valves ensure that the flow of blood goes only towards the heart.

the greater the amount of blood needed to nourish the hard-working muscles. Gravity helps to drain areas which are above the level of the heart but the main mechanism for returning the blood from the tissues is the muscle pump.

As the name suggests, muscles are at the centre of this

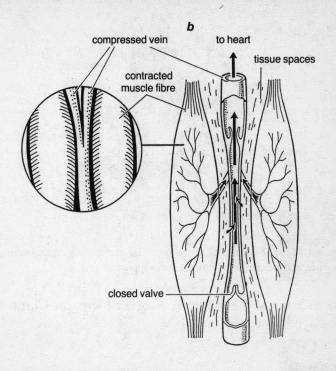

b

compressed vein

to heart

tissue spaces

contracted
muscle fibre

closed valve

pumping mechanism. Figure 1.10*b* shows that when a muscle contracts it becomes tight, thus driving the blood out of it and into the veins. Non-return valves ensure that the flow is in one direction only – towards the heart. Furthermore, a vital function of the muscle pump is that as the contracting muscles expand they also put pressure on the adjacent tissues which drives the tissue fluid out from the tissues and back into the bloodstream. This compresses the veins as well, driving the fluid in them back to the heart.

Later we will look at how back problems can interfere with the action of the muscle pump, leading to pain and

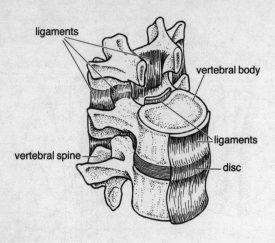

Figure 1.11 The ligaments of the spine are very strong, surrounding the discs and vertebrae to protect and support.

also to many of the problems associated with the Chronic Back Syndrome.

Ligaments

These run as large bands up and down the spinal column and, as figure 1.11 shows, they also wrap around the small joints. Ligaments give the spinal column strength, hold the bones together and generally act in a supportive way. They could be described as doorstops, limiting excessive movement and preventing dislocation of both the large and small joints, and of the vertebrae.

Ligaments are made up of bands of fibrous tissue, which is relatively primitive. Cells in tissues usually start life as simple structures which become more and more complex as they become fully developed and able to perform the function of the particular tissue they make up. Some tissues, however, such as fibrous tissue, which makes up the

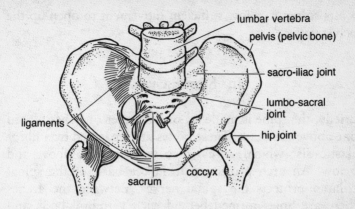

Figure 1.12 The sacro-iliac joints, between the sacrum and the pelvis.

ligaments, have little function other than support so the cells remain simple. The ability to repair or reproduce is usually greatest in the simple cells and least in the most complex ones. So, although the fibrous tissues which make up the ligaments can be torn in a severe injury, their powers of repair are quite considerable and they rarely sustain any lasting damage.

Sacro-iliac joints

As figure 1.12 shows, the sacro-iliac joints are large flattish joints which separate the sacrum from the iliac bones. They are not moving joints, like the knee or shoulder joints, but a somewhat irregular gap between the sacrum (the fused lower part of the spinal column) and the ilium (one of the bones which, fused together, form the complete pelvic basin). These joints probably do not move at all – or if they do, very very little. The only occasion upon which they come into their own is during childbirth and pregnancy when the powerful ligaments attached to the joints soften to allow sufficient movement to open up the pelvic gap.

In Summary . . .

Briefly, the spine is made up of a number of bones placed one above the other. These bones are separated by a fibro-elastic disc which is welded to the vertebrae above and below. An arch projecting from the back of the spinal column protects the spinal nerves. Between the arches there are holes formed behind each vertebral body and these are the neural canals through which the spinal nerves pass.

The floor of these canals is largely made up of facet joints on either side which, with the discs, separate one vertebra from another. These facet joints act like a natural corset to limit the movement and stabilize the back. The vertebrae form such strong and stable interlocking structures that it is very difficult for a vertebra to be displaced unless the injury also fractures a bone.

The large and adequate muscles in the back maintain the posture of the spine and are also responsible for performing and controlling the various movements.

Finally, there are ligaments which run up and down the whole spinal column and also surround the little joints, giving added stability and further helping to strengthen the spine.

In Praise of the Spinal Column

The spinal column is very well adapted for the job it has to do. Indeed, I find it hard to understand the common criticism that the back cannot cope with the upright life we now lead. Many people believe the back was better suited for our primitive life as four-legged animals and that we would suffer far less back trouble if we were antelopes chasing around on all fours. However, it is worth mentioning here that these animals may also suffer back problems. I have seen many dogs and horses with backs as bad as any human.

The common painful back is not a result of faults in the design of the back as is often suggested but by the stress we now impose on it through our present, everyday activities. The back performs its function admirably, providing a firm but flexible base for the maintenance of our shape, for the attachment of muscles and for the protection of vital structures, especially the spinal cord. It is not, however, able to cope with the type of injury inflicted on it by modern life: slipping and falling on to hard, man-made surfaces; the falls and compressional injuries in games such as rugby football; the somewhat more spectacular damage incurred in a skiing accident or falling down stairs; and the altogether different injuries resulting from falling from a horse or being involved in a car accident.

It does not help that most of us take little exercise to keep the circulation going, and spend a lot of time sitting – a condition less favourable to the back. Business, domestic and financial worries, as we shall see later, also place an unnatural strain on our resources. We eat foods that may disagree with our system. Certain foods such as milk and other dairy products, or white flour and additives, can cause a reaction in some people that increases any inflammation in the body – wherever it may be present – and this considerably aggravates back trouble. Finally, in the West we tend to over-eat, which puts yet another load on our skeletal system.

Despite all this, the body is usually able to cope – as long as it remains uninjured. The back is so beautifully formed that I believe it is impossible to blame the mechanics of the spinal column for back pain. In the following chapters we will look at the real causes of back problems.

2

YOUR PAINFUL BACK

*The cause of recurrent
chronic back pain*

The experts tend to agree on the causes and management of the well-recognized and diagnosable diseases of the spine such as tumours, ankylosing spondylitis (where the vertebrae gradually become stiff, fixed and painful with an associated arthritis of the hips), Paget's disease (a thickening of the bones), fractures and spondylolisthesis (where one vertebra slips forward on another). However, the majority of those troubled by back pain do not suffer from any of these specific illnesses and they are therefore grouped as having non-specific back pain. For patients who have nothing very definite to explain their back pain, the answers are as varied as they are vague.

Confusion and Controversy

There must be more controversy about the cause of recurrent attacks of non-specific back pain than almost any other subject in medicine. There is a saying that if you go to ten different consultants, you will get ten different opinions; and that's probably true. The medical profession is likely to suggest a number of reasons for non-specific back pain, including protruding or ruptured discs, wear, strained muscles or ligaments, a strained or displaced sacro-iliac joint, and posture. Many also believe that back pain is due to psychological causes (see Chapter Three).

Alternative practitioners have their own theories, depending on their particular discipline. The osteopath and chiropractor will blame displaced or misaligned vertebrae, displaced discs and back strain. Relaxation therapists blame the patient's posture. Others say the cause of back pain is strained muscles, ligaments, discs, etc., as a result of carrying heavy weights or lifting objects in an ill-advised way. Some people believe diet is at the root of the problem; others blame worry and mental stress.

Now I am about to add my own theory, without adding to the confusion. As a chronic back pain sufferer you will find the theory makes sense and you can easily identify with my explanation. In this chapter I shall use this theory to explain how pain comes about, why it is intermittent and also to show that the underlying cause has a number of other effects on the body.

THAT OLD INJURY

In virtually every patient I have seen with chronic or recurring back pain there is a history of an injury which involved a sharp jolt, jerk or twist such as a hard rugby tackle, falling off a horse, down stairs, or a car accident some years before. It is my belief that these injuries are the cause of back problems. Many of my patients find this difficult to understand at first. Indeed, many have put the initial injury so far in the past they need a lot of prompting to recall what actually happened.

> Jim, thirty-seven, had been complaining of pain in the lumbar region on and off for about seven years. He had no idea what had brought it on. When the pain first started it was an inconveniencing ache. After a while, however, it

became more frequent and more severe. Over the years he noticed that his back was often uncomfortable on rising from bed, when getting up after sitting for any period of time and after prolonged standing. Driving a car had become difficult as he felt sharp pain after about only half an hour.

On examination I felt reasonably sure that the back trouble was caused by an old injury. Jim couldn't remember any such injury, but when I asked his wife she recalled an incident about twelve years before, when he'd fallen down ten stairs. Jim had undergone treatment for the original bruising but he had put the episode completely out of his mind.

How could I be so confident that Jim's past injury was the cause of intermittent back pain? After all, he had been free of pain for five years before he felt any symptoms. To explain I would like to look at the five different basic forms of illness in humans and discuss these forms of illness in relation to the painful back syndrome. By a process of elimination we can see why injury is almost certainly the culprit.

- **Congenital problems**, such as an extra or split vertebrae, are malformations present at birth. They are usually fairly easy to diagnose and are likely to cause trouble from an early age. There is little chance of them starting to cause symptoms later in life, which is when most back trouble begins. Most congenital problems show in an X-ray. In general, they are unlikely to be involved in the type of back pain we are looking at now.
- **Infections** are caused by bacteria or occasionally a virus and have their own definite signs and symptoms. The patient may notice that the area becomes hot and pulsates; there is often swelling, pain and

loss of function. Infections will often show up on an X-ray, and cause the patient to feel unwell and possibly to have a temperature. They may alter the blood count, and a blood sample will then indicate any infection. Infections usually only come on rapidly, and last a short while. Longer-lasting ones become walled in and can be readily diagnosed. Infections are either rapidly cleared as the body's defences overcome them, or they can be treated with an appropriate drug. Very rarely they can be surgically removed. It is not difficult to recognize infections. They would be relatively sudden in onset, unlikely to linger for years and have a predictable end. Infections can usually be eliminated as a cause for this kind of back pain.

- **Tumours and Growths** are usually fairly easy to diagnose. Once the pain has started, there are seldom remissions, especially after a few weeks, and the intensity increases steadily with the onset of time. Growths in the spine are often secondary to a tumour elsewhere and would almost certainly be diagnosed in the initial stages – long before the back pain starts. Persistent intermittent back trouble over many years would almost never be due to tumours or growths so these can also be eliminated as possible causes.

- **Degenerative conditions** are often blamed for causing the back pain syndrome. People are led to believe that back pain is just another part of getting old. I am adamant that this is not so. Ageing and degeneration are quite different processes. Just because you are advancing in years does not mean you or your back are wearing out. When patients of sixty plus are successfully treated they remain free of pain for many, many years.

Because ageing is so often blamed for non-specific back pain, it's important that we take a closer look at its components, and their effects on the back.

Ageing

Ageing is a physiological change where tissues become less efficient and virile. This process is designed to end in death. It is Nature's way of making continuous replacement possible and so allowing for natural selection to continue to improve the species as time goes by. As a slowing down of the repair mechanism takes place with age so the actual performance of the person lessens. The level of wear is always matched by the ability to repair.

Degeneration only occurs under extreme circumstances. It happens when tissues are subjected to protracted excessive strain or when the repair mechanism becomes defective and the tissues involved cannot keep pace with normal wear and tear. The body may attempt to repair the area but the efforts are usually fruitless, as nothing can be done to stop degeneration under these circumstances. Under normal conditions tissues do not degenerate. There is no reason to suppose that the back is any different to the rest of the body.

Many doctors believe that the changes they see in X-rays are caused by degeneration or wear. One of the main changes is an increase in the density and size of bone, especially at joint margins. I believe this is usually due to a compensatory strengthening reaction to the considerable pressure put on the spine by the protective spasms of the muscles, as a result of an injury usually many years before. The spasm is a contraction of the muscles caused by the bruising of the facet joints, and is intended to stiffen the back to give these joints a rest. It has nothing to do with degeneration.

Bone is a living tissue which is permanently readjusting and adapting itself to any change in need or circumstance. A porter constantly carrying heavy loads would get stronger and denser bones in his legs. Similarly, if the pressure of the muscle spasm is putting a great strain on a joint surface then it would be expected to enlarge to meet the challenge. Unfortunately, the extra bone around the edge of a joint is not well formed and is usually irregular in shape.

Another change often apparent in X-rays is a narrowing of the spaces between the vertebrae. Again, this is not usually caused by degeneration of the discs but by the pressure from the protective spasm which compresses them. As both these changes are a normal reaction to the pressure brought about by a spasm, they would not in themselves cause pain. This is borne out by the fact that the degree or extent of *changes* in X-ray pictures bears almost no relationship to the amount or severity of pain. On a number of occasions X-rays taken of organs such as the kidneys, which have the same focus as the spine, and which therefore also show up clearly in the X-rays, have shown very advanced changes in the spine. Yet the patients deny back pain. Similarly, a number of the very worst back sufferers whom I have seen have had completely normal X-rays.

These are some of the reasons why I do not accept that degeneration is the usual cause of the back pain syndrome.

- **Injury** is the last of the groups of pathological processes. In almost all cases – the other groups of illness having been eliminated – the cause of recurrent, chronic back pain is found in this group. In many cases, like Jim's, there is a long quiescent period after the immediate effects of the original injury have settled before the patient first suffers pain. Often there is a second and sometimes quite minor injury that will start the pain.

Susan, forty-three, was strong, athletic and keen on sports. When she came to see me a year ago she was in so much pain she could hardly move. She was very perplexed about the cause of her suffering. She said she had never had any real trouble with her back, although she did feel a little stiff after long car journeys. Then quite out of the blue she'd had a sudden attack of pain.

Her story is a common one. She had come home from a holiday abroad during which, of course, there was a considerable amount of sedentary travelling and carrying of heavy cases. When she arrived home she went into the kitchen to make herself a cup of tea. She leaned forward to lift a cup from the shelf and was seized by agonizing pain in the lumbar region. The pain didn't respond to bed rest, pain killers and later to anti-inflammatory drugs.

After four days, she was brought, with some difficulty, to see me. She was under the impression that reaching for the cup was the cause of the pain but could not understand why. Examination was difficult as movement was so painful, but I could feel the muscle spasm and see that the normal lumbar curve of her back was flattened. This gave me enough evidence to suspect that the real trouble was not due to the stretching action but to an injury sustained some years previously when she had probably slipped and sat down hard. Reaching for the cup had merely been the precipitating factor in the onset of pain.

When this was suggested, Susan remembered an accident on a skiing holiday six years previously when she had slipped on the ice outside her hotel in Switzerland and fallen on her bottom. She was a little shaken up at the time but had soon recovered and was able to finish the skiing holiday without any problems. Indeed, she felt pleased that she had done herself no serious damage. Once the initial discomfort had passed, there were no symptoms and she put the incident to the back of her mind.

It was only when Susan felt the sudden cramp in her back muscles that she was aware she still had trouble. The previous jolt had caused a wave of pressure up her spine compressing the discs and thus jolting the facet joints and bruising them (see figure 2.1). Although there had been no symptoms for many years, the underlying problem remained and the stretching action of reaching for the cup had sparked off the pain. We will now look at why this minor incident precipitated the agonizing attack.

The last straw

It is understandable that Susan should put the blame for the pain on stretching for the cup. This was, after all, her first experience of acute back pain. Similarly, many sufferers believe that their pain is due to straining their backs by lifting or trying to lift a heavy weight – usually a heavy suitcase or piece of furniture – or by pushing a car. A common tale is that they were trying to push a car when suddenly there was a 'click' in the back and they were immediately in agony.

Personally, I doubt that a voluntary effort such as lifting or straining could cause a back injury. If you are straining unsuccessfully to unscrew a jam jar top, do you worry that you might damage the muscles in your forearm and hand? Of course not. You can either undo it, or you can't. You don't expect to be laid up in bed for days with a painful forearm simply because you tried. So why should you expect dramatic problems if you put any other part of the body to the limit of muscular effort? It seems strange that it should be so universally agreed that the back alone will suffer under these circumstances. As we have already

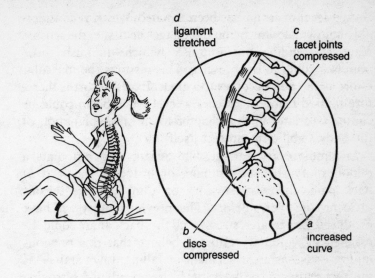

Figure 2.1 The effect of a blow to the spine. At point *a*, the spine has increased its curve to absorb the shock; *b* shows the compression of the discs (greatest at the lower end); *c* indicates how the blow affects the facet joints, which limit movement, and *d* illustrates the stretched ligament.

seen in the previous chapter, the back is particularly well adapted to the work it has to do.

The impossibility of this commonly held belief is also borne out by looking at the physiology of the skeletal system. Our muscles, tendons, ligaments and joints all have a large number of sensors which measure and monitor every function of every tissue. There are many different types of sensor – each one with a particular function such as measuring blood pressure, body temperature, the amount a joint is bent and skin sensations. One type detects the pulling strain on the tissue. These sensors work to protect the area from self-inflicted damage. Once a certain level of strain has been reached, which is considerably below that which could damage the tissue, the sensors react by sending out impulses which diminish those impulses going to the muscles. This restricts the muscular effort as the pull becomes too great. Excess effort is therefore limited before it reaches a level when harm could be caused (see later in this chapter for a full explanation of the body's ability to protect itself).

In almost every patient, like Susan, who pinpoints a minor injury such as straining or lifting as the start of back pain, there is a history of a much more serious incident some years before. This previous injury will have produced far greater stresses in the back than could be reached by voluntary effort. I believe that this previous injury – such as a car accident or falling down stairs – is the real cause of the back problem and that the trouble then lies latent for a period of time. You notice it for the first time when you are involved in a much less traumatic activity.

A SHOCK TO THE SYSTEM

If an old injury is the cause of back problems, we must now examine the possible effects of that injury. What does it do to the back? Why does it cause intermittent pain? Why does the pain vary so much in its severity? Why is there so often a long, symptomless period before a sudden attack of pain? What is the progress of events? To explain, let us consider the example of someone who falls a short distance and sits down very heavily on a hard floor. Figure 2.1 illustrates damage done by this kind of injury. Patricia had had just such an accident.

Patricia came to see me when she was thirty-two. She said she had suffered back trouble on and off since she was in her teens. In the last two or three years it had been ruining her life. Whatever she did was painful. Unlike so many patients she could vividly recall the initial injury that sparked the problem. She was fifteen and enjoying a disco with a new boyfriend. After a particularly energetic dance, he suggested they have a drink.

Now this practical joker thought he'd try a trick on Patricia. He pulled up a chair for her but just as she was about to sit down he yanked it away. She went crashing on to the dance floor, giving her back a very nasty bump. Needless to say she didn't think it was at all funny. The boyfriend didn't last long, but the problem lingered on.

An injury such as Susan's or Patricia's results in:

1. increased flexion of the normal curves of the back particularly the lumbar curve which is the first to be affected by the blow;
2. a compressional force directly through the vertebrae and discs;
3. a hard jolt to the lumbo-sacral joint at the base of the spine and the sacro-iliac joints between the spine and the pelvis;
4. sharp stretching of the ligaments and possibly the muscles, both of which may be torn; and
5. bruising of the facet joints whose primary function is to stabilize one vertebra to the next and to limit movement in nearly all directions.

WHEN NATURE DOESN'T KNOW BEST

Nature responds to the bruising of any joint in the body by trying to protect and help it repair itself. The emergency repair mechanism, or the inflammatory reaction, ensures that the blood supply is greatly increased to the affected tissues, thus bringing extra oxygen and nutrients. In addition, the sensors in the joint, which are specially designed to detect bruising and inflammation, will send impulses along a nerve to the spinal cord. There, the impulses cross directly to the motor nerves and via them to the muscles which move the joint. These impulses put the muscles across the joint into a protective contraction called a spasm. The level of the spasm is controlled by the number of impulses coming from the bruised joint. It follows then that the more severe the bruising, the stronger the contraction.

Protective spasm

The spasm is a perfectly normal contraction of the muscle, controlled by the nerves. It is our bodies' way of promoting repair of the bruising and we are completely unaware of it occurring. The idea is that the spasm acts as a kind of splint or corset. By stiffening the joint to prevent or limit movement, the joint surfaces should be given a recuperative rest.

Unlike an agonizing muscle cramp, there are no symptoms when a muscle is in spasm. While a spasm is a controlled contraction sent down the normal nerve route, a cramp is uncontrolled, originating in the muscle itself through some internal fault. The intensity of the pull in a bad cramp is sufficient to produce a pain that has been described as an oversized spear stuck in the area. A spasm is symptomless.

Figure 2.2 In diagram *a*, a voluntary muscle contraction, the movement is started in the brain, travelling down the spinal cord, arriving at the junction box at the correct level in the spinal cord, and passing from the junction box to the muscle, causing it to contract. In diagram *b*, a muscle spasm, the impulses start in a bruised facet joint and they pass to the junction box, via the same nerve, causing an identical contraction.

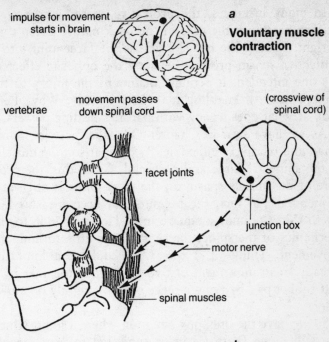

impulse for movement starts in brain

a
Voluntary muscle contraction

movement passes down spinal cord

(crossview of spinal cord)

vertebrae

facet joints

junction box

motor nerve

spinal muscles

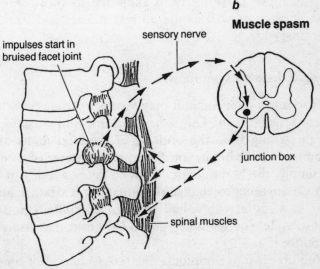

b
Muscle spasm

sensory nerve

impulses start in bruised facet joint

junction box

spinal muscles

49

In many instances, the protective spasm works well. Unfortunately, in the case of the back nature doesn't get it right. Putting the muscles across the facet joint into a protective spasm produces exactly the opposite effect to the one intended. It actually maintains the injury to the joint instead of enabling it to heal quickly. Why? Let's look at what goes wrong with nature's healing powers.

As we have seen in Chapter One, the facet joints are small and relatively inflexible. By comparison the muscles in the spine are large and powerful. Given this, the pressure of the muscle spasm on the facet joints is obviously tremendous. In fact, the pressure has been measured at up to thirty pounds a square inch. However, due to the mechanics of the spine, the spasm does little to limit the movement. Think of it this way, could you limit the already small movement of two tins joined together by a soft rubber pad by tying a piece of string tightly on either side?

So we have the unhappy situation where a joint, which can still move fairly freely, is subjected to considerable extra pressure as well as the normal stresses and strains of ordinary life.

Why are there no symptoms?

With so much happening, it may seem surprising that the patient feels no pain. This is because any mild sensations of pain arising from the bruising of the facet joints are suppressed by the brain, you are no longer aware of them. Put simply, the brain doesn't want to know about it if it can't do anything to change the situation. It's rather like being in a room with a bad smell or continuous noise. After a while, you gradually get so used to it that you do not notice it at all.

With no obvious symptoms over a long period of time,

it's not surprising that most patients believe their backs have made a full recovery. Indeed, as I was going through a batch of several hundred case histories recently I found that there was an average of eleven years from an original injury to the first symptoms arising.

As no pain is experienced during this time, other signs are needed to demonstrate that there is trouble still present in the spine. One is that the protective spasm of the muscles makes them feel very firm and the other is that the pull of the muscles often alters the normal curve of the back. Although patients are not aware of the spasm, it can readily be detected because it is so firm to touch. Try contracting the muscles of your arm; feel the firmness. That is what I am looking for when I examine a patient by palpation (diagnosis by touch). To show you just how evident a spasm is on touch, I would like to relate the story of a skiing friend of mine:

Leo phoned me a few years ago to say that his back was troubling him a great deal. On examination I diagnosed his trouble as being due to an old injury, mainly because I could feel the firm protective spasm of the back muscles. After several sessions of treatment he was pain-free and the spasm had almost completely gone.

Two years later Leo and his wife invited me to a dinner party during which he complained that his back was as bad as it had been before he came to see me. Being rather surprised by this, I asked to have a quick look at his back and we retired to another room. When I felt his back I found there was a great deal of recent bruising but very little evidence of the firm protective spasm I had originally treated. I explained that this was not the original problem but a fairly recent injury to his back.

Leo denied that he had injured his back recently, but while I was still brooding over the problem, our hostess proudly switched on a video of her husband getting his gold medal at skiing. It was quite a revelation.

At one moment when Leo was coming down the mountan at sixty miles per hour there was a minor atomic explosion and, after a cloud of snow had settled, there was no sign of him or his skis. It was lucky, he said, that they were taking the video or he wouldn't have been noticed so quickly. He had been knocked out and fallen down an eight-foot-deep hole with all the snow on top of him. And this was the man who said he had not injured his back since I had last treated him!

At this point I'd like to recap by using the illustration of another patient:

> Dorothy, a thirty-eight-year-old mother, came to see me five years ago. She had fallen downstairs twenty years before and had hurt herself but felt fortunate there was no serious injury. She had noticed that her back ached after long car journeys or sitting for any length of time but as this went away so quickly she did not worry about it. Then, seven years ago, while she was leaning over the bath and bathing her child, her back went 'click'. It was agony at the time and had remained troublesome.
>
> Dorothy tried osteopathy, physiotherapy, acupuncture and drugs. Some were helpful but just for a short time. She complained of bad pain in the lumbar region and occasionally it was so severe it radiated down the leg.
>
> As I examined her back I could feel the distinct spasm of the paravertebral muscles (the ones that run up and down the back between the vertebrae) from the lower half of the thoracic spine to the low lumbar region particularly in the mid-lumber region. She had seven visits by which time the spasm had largely gone. She has been free of back trouble ever since.

Let us look at what happened to Dorothy's back when

she fell downstairs all those years ago. Her spine received a blow and bruising to the facet joints, and nature tried to protect the joints and promote healing in its usual way by putting the muscles into spasm. However, the pressure on these joints was so strong that it maintained the injury. For many years Dorothy was unaware that she had any problem. Then the bathtime incident sparked off the pain by stretching and overworking the muscles, causing them to go into a painful cramp.

This delay in the appearance of the symptoms can give rise to problems of obtaining compensation for injuries sustained, for example, at work or in a car accident. During the course of my work I am called upon to give evidence in court cases where there is some dispute as to the reason for the current pain and the disruption to everyday activities experienced by the sufferer. In many such cases I have had to satisfy the court that it was actually the injury which occurred many years before which was at the root of the problem. Compensation has been awarded accordingly.

LEADING UP TO AN ATTACK

The next question we must ask is why, after such a long, trouble-free period, patients have an attack of pain followed by intermittent attacks. To answer this, we need to study the sequence of events that leads from the silent stage to the attack of pain. Hopefully the ensuing diagrams will help clarify my explanation of this rather complex process. You may also like to refer back to the previous chapter.

One of the functions of the muscles is the part they play in the circulation of the blood. At this point let me once again clarify the common misapprehension that the heart pumps the blood round and round the body, like the pump

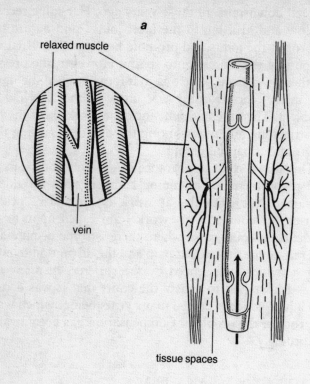

Figure 2.3 In diagram *a*, the thin, relaxed muscle exerts little pressure, allowing the veins and tissue spaces to fill. In diagram *b*, however, you can see how the hard, contracting muscle exerts pressure. It squeezes the blood back to the heart, the valves ensuring one-way flow.

in a domestic central heating system. As we noted earlier, this is not so. In the body, the blood pressure is due to the resistance to its flow from the minute arterioles. When it flows through them into the capillaries and into the tissues it is at a low pressure.

Imagine a heating system that had radiators made of

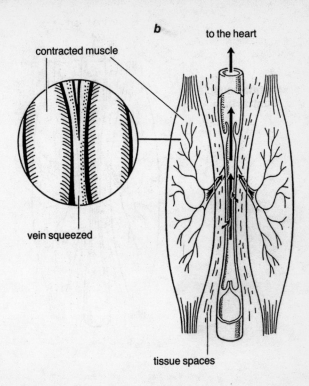

thin latex rubber. The fluid would flow into them, expanding them and, if we ignored the elastic property of the rubber, have no force left to return the fluid into the pipes and back to the heart. The radiators would need to be squeezed to push the fluid out of them and into the pipes leading back to the pump. They would then need to be relaxed to enable re-filling, and then be squeezed again. As the return pipes have non-return valves this results in a pumping effect to complete the second half of the circulation from the tissues – along the veins and back to the heart.

In the body, it is the muscles which administer the

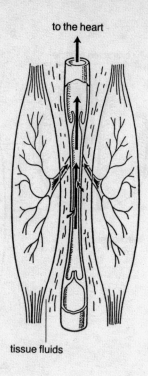

to the heart

a

**normal muscle
contraction**

tissue fluids

Figure 2.4 Diagram *a* illustrates a normal contraction, which allows fluid to circulate by squeezing the veins and tissue spaces. In diagram *b*, the muscle in spasm is permanently contracted, and this does not allow the veins to refill – or to be squeezed out again. The pumping action becomes slower and slower as the tissue fluids clog and collect in the tissue spaces.

squeeze and so provide the force required to pump it on. Every time a muscle contracts it tightens and squeezes out blood – first into tiny veins and then into bigger and bigger ones. Non-return valves make this a one-way traffic system back to the heart. The contracted muscle also squeezes

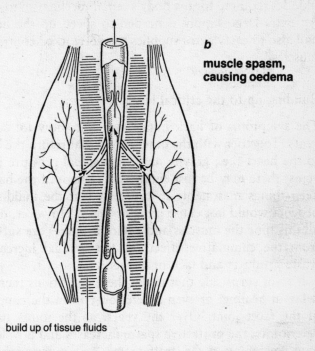

b

**muscle spasm,
causing oedema**

build up of tissue fluids

the nearby tissues. The pumping effect therefore spreads beyond the muscles to the adjacent tissues (see figure 2.3).

When a muscle is in spasm following an injury, the alternate relaxation and contraction is interfered with. The spasm increases the supply of blood to the muscles to cope with the extra work caused by the permanent contraction, but reduces the efficiency of the muscle pump. Fluid diffuses out of the blood and builds up in the tissue spaces. This causes water-logging in the tissue spaces creating a situation rather like a traffic jam. This extra fluid in the tissues is called oedema (see figure 2.4b).

This 'traffic jam' situation also means that there is a less effective blood supply in precisely the area where the most blood is required for the body's repair mechanism to work. An extra-large supply is needed to speed up the healing and also to carry extra supplies to overworked contracting muscles.

Building up to the critical level

The symptoms of back injury may not show for several years. Together with the other forces that return the blood to the heart (i.e., gravity and the residual pressure in the veins) there may be just enough movement of the back to keep things reasonably in order so that the build-up of oedema would not cause a major upset. However, during all this time the muscles and adjacent tissues are suffering from the cumulative effects of the gradual increase in waste products and lack of oxygen.

It's not surprising that under these conditions there is a delay in healing, or even a deterioration in the condition of the facet joint. Over the years, as the joints further deteriorate, the protective spasm increases and is followed by a worsening of the 'traffic jam'. As a muscle spasm is a normal contraction, the patient does not feel any pain at this time, but finally, the situation reaches such a critical point that – due to lack of oxygen and a build-up of waste products – the muscle can no longer function normally and goes into a cramp. This is an abnormal contraction generated in the muscle itself and this is what produces pain. If only a few of the thousands of muscle fibres are affected then the patient will feel a slight ache. If more fibres are affected then the pain is proportionally greater; if the whole muscle is in cramp, then the pain is agonizing.

THE ONSET OF PAIN

The three common precipitating factors of pain are as follows.

- **Muscular effort.** This kind of strain can be quick and intense, such as lifting a heavy weight, or less arduous but more prolonged, such as digging the garden. Both cause an increase of blood circulating to the working muscles to supply the extra oxygen required and remove the waste products. There is a critical point when, due to the lack of oxygen and the build-up of waste products, the muscles go into cramp.

- **Complete rest.** Not surprisingly, this diminishes the workings of the muscle pump. If the muscle is already in spasm, rest will further reduce the effect of the muscle pump to an inadequate level. There comes a point when the utilization of oxygen and the production of waste products give rise to the conditions for a cramp.

- **Stretching the muscle.** A bending or twisting movement often sets off pain. The stretching raises the pressure in the muscle, which already has excessive fluid in it, and this causes the monitoring sensors in the muscles to send out excessive impulses, which lead to a violent correcting contraction, trying to oppose the stretching and restore the muscle to its normal length. This has the same effect as the quick and intense muscular effort considered above and can cause an immediate cramp. Stretching under slow, controlled conditions can be beneficial to people with back trouble as this activates the muscle pump. However, if the movement is sharp then the muscles react badly to it by becoming much nearer the point when they will go into a cramp.

REACHING CRISIS POINT

The final question we must address in this chapter is why there can be such a difference in the severity of the incident that sets off the pain. Why does one person suffer an attack of pain doing something as seemingly effortless as bending to tie her shoelaces while someone else only reaches crisis level when she single-handedly reorganizes the furniture in the lounge.

Much depends on the condition of the muscle and how far away it is from the trigger point of the crisis. If it is extremely close to the critical point, with the build-up of waste products and lack of oxygen, then, as in a great number of my patients, only a minor strain such as the movement of leaning forward slightly to look in a mirror is necessary to produce the cramp. If the muscles are not yet near crisis point with moderate oxygen reserves and not too excessive a build-up of waste, the patient might need a very big muscular effort – like trying to push a car – for the tremendous increase in oxygen requirements and the build-up of waste products to bridge the gap, putting the muscles into a sudden cramp.

Lastly, there is the very common situation of quite energetic work, which causes considerable strain on the patient's back and may have taken quite a long time. Digging in the garden or, as we mentioned above, re-arranging the furniture, may well involve sufficient muscular movement in the back to keep reasonable circulation going. The increased muscular effort will, however, result in a considerable increase in the overall blood supply and this continues after the actual work is finished – perhaps when the person is resting or watching television.

This causes a steady increase in the tissue fluid and local pressure, making it much more difficult to maintain the circulation in the tissues. The build-up of waste products and the lack of oxygen gradually produces a crisis in the muscles and the patient has the paradox of pain – not at the time of the effort – but some time afterwards.

You may now have found that my explanation for the cause of back pain fits your particular problem. In Chapter Four we will look at specific types of back pain, but before continuing, I would like to devote the next chapter to answering some of the questions most frequently asked by my patients.

3

YOUR BACK IN QUESTION

*Clear answers to
common queries*

This chapter uses my theory of the cause of non-specific back pain to offer logical explanations to the questions that puzzle so many people who suffer from this intermittently. The most commonly asked questions are answered here.

Why is my back so often at its worst first thing in the morning?

It seems strange to many people that their backs should be troublesome when they've been in bed for some time. This is the very time you would expect it to be well rested, and after all, doctors so often advise bed rest for bad backs. However, rest actually *aggravates* the underlying problem.

As we have seen in the previous chapter, when a muscle is in spasm there is an increased supply of blood to the muscles and tissues, but the muscle pump does not work efficiently. Extra fluid, or oedema, builds up, leading to an increase in waste products and oxygen deficiency. When you are asleep your muscle pump is at an all-time low. Oedema accumulates until it reaches a maximum level which, from the experiences of my patients, seems to be around three in the morning or later. They are often woken by the pain. The worst moment is often experienced when the sufferer tries to get out of bed. By this time even slight muscular effort is enough to cause a cramp.

When you get up and move around some of the fluid is squeezed out of the tissues, improving the circulation, and the likelihood of a painful cramp diminishes. In a short time, the back can become symptom-free and comfortable.

Why is it that I can manage a fairly energetic task such as digging in the garden and not feel any pain, only to experience agony once I sit down.

A curious fact, you may say, but it makes sense when you think about it. While you are gardening, the movement is sufficient to squeeze out enough blood – despite the increased blood supply to the muscles brought about by the effort – to keep them below the threshold of pain. However, the increased blood supply produced by the extra muscular effort does not immediately diminish when the digging stops. It continues for some hours after the actual work is finished and floods out of the muscles since, when the body is at rest, the pumping effect is now greatly reduced. So later in the day, or even the next one, you experience pain when you are simply seated watching television or possibly relaxing in bed.

Why does exercise help?

Patients often extol the benefits of exercise. A daily swim or gentle work-out is the ticket to a pain-free life. The trouble is that once regular exercise ceases, the intermittent pain starts again.

> Charles was twenty when he was involved in a car accident. He suffered a mild whiplash injury but the symptoms disappeared very rapidly, without any treatment. He was

63

badly shaken up at the time. Ten years later, he felt a 'click' in his back as he picked up his three-year-old daughter. He sought help from an osteopath, who relieved him of the pain, but from then on Charles started to complain of painful twinges in his back when he got up in the morning and after long journeys.

On the advice of a friend, Charles took up yoga. He was overjoyed at how much it helped ease the aches and pains. He kept it up for nearly three years and was relatively symptom-free during this time. Then he got a job promotion which meant a busy schedule and no time for yoga. Only a month after stopping the regular activity he started to experience pain in his back again.

Exercise may keep you out of pain but it often does little to correct the basic problem. It works by activating the muscle pump and so decreasing the likelihood of the muscle going into a cramp. The muscles are prevented from turning a constant protective spasm into a cramp by the regular replenishment of exercise. Once the exercise stops, it does not take long for the muscles to move into a critical state.

Does age affect back problems?

I am commonly asked whether age makes any difference to the severity of back trouble. 'Can you help my mother? She is nearly eighty and has been told she is now too old for treatment to be able to work', is one example. In my experience, people of a mature age respond to treatment more quickly and easily than most other age groups. By the time a person reaches the age of sixty-five his or her muscles begin to weaken and they probably stress themselves less. It follows that the spasm could also be weaker. In many cases the back undergoes a spontaneous improvement around this time.

Gladys, aged seventy-three, came to see me because she had a painful right knee. She had damaged it about six months previously. It had not recovered and was actually slowly deteriorating. It was the only joint in her body to be affected so I asked her, among other things, whether she had had back trouble. She said that she had suffered back pain on and off for many years but that in the last five years she'd had much less pain and had more or less forgotten about her back. The telltale spasm could be felt, and after it had been treated, her knee made a slow but good recovery.

Young people often seem to be able to cope with an injury without suffering any pain for many years. This is probably because they have resilient repair mechanisms and usually move about a great deal, even though the muscles are in spasm. Then, when they reach their twenties or thirties and they are less actively involved in sport, their repair mechanisms stop doing such a good job. The 'traffic-jam' situation in the back begins to worsen and the person may well start suffering episodes of pain. It is also possible that the childhood aches and pains which adults so readily label 'growing pains' are actually the start of back trouble.

Will I get better quicker if I am very fit?

No. The level of fitness and general muscle strength of the sufferer have a profound effect on the course of the treatment, but in exactly the opposite way to what you'd expect. In an extremely fit person, spasm is tremendous. These people may experience pain more easily and the pain may be more severe. Many tough men have been brought to tears by the pain.

One of the most worrying patients that I have ever treated

was a man who had recently been the world's non-Japanese Judo champion. He was about five feet, eight inches tall and seemed about the same width. The muscles in his back were absolutely enormous and felt as big as an average person's thigh. He had suffered back trouble for some years and had attacks of extremely severe pain.

I was almost worn out every time I treated him because the spasm of his back produced a resistance that must have been two or three times more than an average person's back. When I had got him, say, seventy-five per cent better, the spasm or pressure of the back muscles on the joints was still probably as great as that of a less fit person at their worst. The number of treatments that he needed for a full recovery was three or four times more than usual.

Why is my back so painful after a long journey?

You may well find that two of the worst things for your back trouble are sitting for long periods in a chair, or – even more disastrous – in a car or airplane. Indeed, a car journey is probably about the most difficult situation that an injured back can be asked to tolerate.

Let us consider what happens to your back when you are immobilized in the sitting position. The back muscles are stretched as the thighs go out at a right angle. A poorly supported back will become more curved, and also stretch the back muscles. In addition, the limited movement diminishes the muscle pump.

Now add the motion of a car. The muscles in your back will have to work hard consistently to keep you upright against the stresses of a motor car in action. When turning corners, the muscles have to resist the trunk lurching sideways; when braking, they must resist the body falling forwards; and, when accelerating, they may have to resist some backward movement.

There will also be little jolts through the spine from the

bumps on the road, which fractionally may increase the bruising of the facet joints and thus the spasm of the back.

It's hardly surprising that a car journey should give rise to problems. However, once the journey is over and you start to move about, the muscle pump is resumed and the trouble soon subsides. For this reason, it is wise to plan a series of short stops on a long journey. Keep the muscle pump activated by taking a little exercise – even walking around the car can be enough.

Is bad posture the cause of back pain?

Most of us can recall countless childhood reprimands for poor posture. You probably make a point of correcting your own children for slouching and stooping. However, as we saw in Chapter One, we have very little voluntary control over our posture. In general, posture is controlled by an automatic mechanism based on the small brain, or cerebellum, which controls repetitive functions in the body. If, say, the body tilts forwards a little in an involuntary movement, this will automatically be corrected by muscles tightening to pull the body back into a normal posture. If, however, the back is injured and some groups of muscle have gone into spasm and thus an increased contraction, it is easy to see that the normal posture can be upset. The curve of the back would either be increased much as the tightening strings on a bow, or, if the opposite group of muscles were affected, then the normal curve would tend to be flattened (see figure 3.1).

Many people believe poor posture leads to back pain, but slouching and stooping are the effect of back trouble rather than the cause. It is important to realize that it is back trouble which gives rise to poor posture and not the reverse. Once the back has been treated and the muscle spasm reduced, then the posture will usually correct itself.

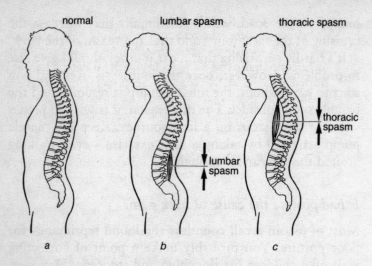

normal   lumbar spasm   thoracic spasm

Figure 3.1 Diagram *a* shows a normal spine, with average posture.
Diagram *b* indicates an increased curve in the lumbar region (lower
back), caused by a spasm there. Diagram *c* illustrates an increased
thoracic curve (upper back), caused by spasm. Note how the curves
in *b* and *c* cause the other curves to increase, as the body attempts to
remain upright.

To illustrate this, we will look at the story of Arabella
who, from the age of twelve, was forced to try every trick
in the book to correct her posture.

Arabella, then a twenty-year-old student, was in absolute
agony when she came to see me many years ago. Two
weeks previously, she had lifted a television and felt a
'click' in her back. She'd also suffered slight pain at the
moment. The next morning she was in severe pain in the
lumbar region which did not respond to bed rest or anti-
inflammatory drugs and painkillers.

When asked about any previous injuries, Arabella
remembered falling off a swing at the age of eight and
bruising her back. It recovered very rapidly, as so often
happens in a child, and did not need treatment. Four years

later, Arabella's parents and teachers started nagging her about her posture. She remembers walking with books on her head, practising endless stretching exercises and fighting a continual battle to keep her back straight. Her back started to ache at the age of seventeen for no particular reason and this was put down to growing pains. She remembers vaguely that she lifted something fairly light and the next day she felt some pain.

Arabella stood with a marked increase of the thoracic curve of the spine (the curve of the spine enclosed by the ribs). She was in too much pain to test movement but on palpation I could feel a severe spasm of the muscles on either side of the lumbar spine and this was also present in decreasing intensity as far as her neck. It took eleven visits in all to get things right but by the end of the treatment she was altogether more comfortable. She also felt better in her general health and her posture improved considerably. After almost fourteen years, Arabella has had no more back trouble. The nagging about her poor deportment has also stopped.

Not everyone is as fortunate as Arabella. If the excessive curve has been present over a long period of time, in some cases the vertebrae can become wedged-shaped to accommodate this. Although the person is free from pain, a slight residual curve remains and becomes the normal posture.

Does anxiety give rise to back problems?

One of my patients once experienced the first agonizing pain in his back when he read a letter informing him that one of his companies had gone bust. Does anxiety bring on back pain, he was keen to know? What is the connection? It is my belief that if and only if a patient has an underlying back problem, then states of anxiety, tension, fright and excitement can indeed be among the factors which produce pain. In some cases, they may even seem to be the only factors involved. To explain my point I would like to consider the subject in some detail.

Although man has been variously civilized for probably twelve thousand years, the fact remains that most of the physiological functions of the body still relate entirely to the primitive state. In those early times, anxiety was generally linked with physical danger, resulting in the subjective sensation which we call fright. This activates a special push-button mechanism called the sympathetic nervous system, which is associated with the adrenalin glands. The body is immediately put into a state of great efficiency for the suspected emergency.

The sensation of fear stimulates the system and the body reacts rather like a ship clearing the decks and getting the guns ready for a fight. In the case of the body it may be flight rather than fight, but either way it must do all that is necessary to increase its chances of survival.

These survival tactics include, amongst others; increasing body temperature through the muscle activity of trembling. Everything works better at a higher temperature (think of a snake whose muscle temperature depends on its environment – it hardly moves when cold but becomes a very quick-moving animal in the hot sunshine). All body functions improve at high temperatures. The pulse speeds up, the blood pressure and blood sugar levels rise, and the blood is re-routed from the skin (which goes white) and stomach (causing butterflies) to the muscles and brain where it will be most required and, in the context of back trouble, the muscles are put into a contraction, ready for action. This makes the muscles work harder and may result in a cramp. This series of 'fight-or-flight' reactions especially apply to the upper muscles of the arm, shoulder girdle and thoracic spine. The lumbar muscles are also involved, but to a lesser extent.

In terms of nature, the time element is minimal. You are either dinner yourself or you have to get your dinner in a relatively short space of time. It is all over very quickly. The sensation of fright or anxiety prepares the body for rapid and efficient action.

In contemporary times, we all suffer anxieties and tensions. They may not require the same urgent response as in primitive days, but they are a form of the same fear and the body automatically reacts. The reaction is much less intense but in our stressful lives it can continue for hours, days, weeks or even months. Under these conditions the increased tension in the muscles can easily be the critical factor in turning a symptomless back into a painful one.

Is back pain psychosomatic?

While I do believe that anxiety and tension can certainly be precipitating factors in the onset of back pain, I am convinced that back trouble is not psychosomatic; although, certainly, many complaints are psychosomatic. Patients, like Judy, whose story follows, have a mental problem which they cannot face. This problem manifests itself in physical symptoms which are usually designed to generate sympathy or change the sufferer's way of life for the better in some way.

Most cases of back-related problems *are* due to damage; however, some psychological cases do exist, like Judy's.

Judy came to me complaining of a very painful knee. Although it had been operated on twice, she said there'd been no improvement. I was not able to find any clinical signs to account for her problems and so I began to ask

71

about any other worries or concerns. After a while she confided that she dreaded having sexual relations with her husband. An ideal excuse presented itself when she had banged her knee on a table six years before, and the pain gave her a substitute for a 'headache'.

As the years went by, her subconscious manufactured the pain for the escape it gave her. She wasn't aware she was doing it. She genuinely believed her knee was in a bad state. I referred her to a psychiatrist and once she faced up to the real problem, her pain vanished.

Judy's pain was psychosomatic. She couldn't cope with a problem and therefore resolved it by suffering physical symptoms. Many doctors believe back pain is psychosomatic. Patients are often told there is no actual physical cause for their pain and they come to me for a second opinion. On examination I always find the pain to be very real and sometimes wonder why the sufferers have not complained more.

The first thing Edna did when she walked into my consulting room was to hand me a letter from her doctor. The letter said that although Edna complained of pain between her shoulders and in the lumbar region, he could find nothing wrong. He said he was only allowing her to come to me because she had insisted so strongly. He stated that her main problem was psychological and that the best thing I could do was to endorse the need for her to go to the psychiatrist that he was recommending.

Edna, a forty-eight-year-old secretary, told me that she had become increasingly tired and low over the last seven years, and that she had started suffering occasional aches in her upper back over this time – especially during and after typing. She had been having treatment with diet and antacids for indigestion for two and a half years, but each time this only gave relief for a few months.

In the last few months the pain had become somewhat

worse and she was now experiencing a new pain around her left chest. She had had physiotherapy with heat mass-age and traction on and off for some time but this only gave temporary relief.

Detailed investigations ruled out heart trouble and no apparent problem could be found, so I conducted my own examination. During the consultation, Edna revealed that she had been involved in a bad fall on a skating rink fifteen years before. I was therefore not surprised to find intense spasm of the spinal muscles. This was particularly obvious in the mid to upper thoracic spine. My examination con-firmed the physical nature of her problem and a very tender fourth thoracic spine pointed to the cause of the chest pain.

After fourteen sessions of treatment with my form of physiotherapy and manipulation to the thoracic spine and muscles, Edna was altogether better.

By their very nature psychosomatic complaints are designed to gain sympathy and attention. Back pain, how-ever, is greeted with laughter or boredom. A painful back is second only to a mother-in-law as a music-hall joke, and if people do not laugh when you complain of your pain then the chances are their eyes will glaze over as they stop listening after the first sentence. People do not feel sorry for back-pain sufferers and the pain certainly does nothing to improve a patient's way of life.

I am satisfied that out of the several thousand people that I have seen with back problems I have yet to meet one with a painful back for psychological reasons.

What is the effect of the weather?

It is often greeted with some amusement if one suggests that the weather has any effect on painful backs and arthritis. Similarly, people laugh when anyone claims he can forecast a change in the weather by the state of his rheumatics. Yet, the fact remains that many back-pain sufferers do actually feel less pain on warm, sunny days or in clear, mountainous climes. Why should this be so? Weather definitely has an effect!

Firstly, I would like to stress that humidity is not usually an influencing factor, as so many people believe. It is a common assumption that when the air is humid there is probably poor evaporation from the surfaces such as the skin, lungs and the nose and throat, which leads to an increase in total body fluid. This, they mistakenly believe, would cause any already inflamed areas to become more swollen and, in the case of joints, more painful.

But humidity is not necessarily a bad thing. After all, we are sent away on a seaside holiday or a cruise as a pick-me-up after an illness or operation. The confusion is not helped by contradictory advertisements in the same magazine – the one claiming to improve the atmosphere in the home by humidifying the air, and another by dehumidifying it. Which one are we supposed to believe?

To put matters straight, let me repeat that humidity is not a factor in back pain; it is the state of electrical charge or ionization of the particles in the air which causes these differences in the level of back pain. In sunny weather the air is predominantly negatively charged. With wind and wet weather, the air becomes more positively charged. The body is unaffected by negatively charged particles, but a positive charge (ions) can cause trouble (see below). An ion is a charged particle of gas; i.e., the air, or particles of pollen or dust. In sunny weather, when the air is charged with negative ions, patients can cope with particles that may cause an allergy. On wet and windy days these same particles may incite an attack of asthma or hay fever.

So let us look at what happens when you breathe the

positive ions into the lungs. The ions pass through the lungs to the blood where they react on the platelets, causing them to secrete a substance called serotonin. It is the serotonin which increases any inflammation and this intensifies any aches and pains. It also makes people feel lethargic, headachy and depressed.

A thunderstorm illustrates my point most dramatically. Before the storm there is a plethora of positive ions and all the symptoms that go with them. Most of us can predict the oncoming storm because we feel a heaviness in ourselves. A few flashes of lightning restore the negative charge and, although the steaming humidity remains the same, people suddenly feel quite different. All the aches, pains and headaches go and everyone feels bright and alert. Ionizers, if of a suitable type and adequate output, can be a great help in the home or place of work. One in the output of an air-conditioning plant can cure the 'sick building syndrome'.

Do weight or height influence back pain?

When no definite cause is known for back pain, then people will blame almost anything they can imagine. Weight and height are common scapegoats – it's because I'm too tall, too short, too fat, too thin. Yet, from my experience, these factors are rarely to blame.

Overweight people are often told that the excess poundage is the cause of their back problem, but this is not often the case. After all, most of us know very overweight people who have no trouble with their backs. Being overweight is not a cause of back pain in itself but if you already have a troublesome back then it may aggravate the situation. The extra weight may alter the curve of your back, thus stretching the muscles. This would increase their workload and also make a cramp more likely. Attacks of pain may occur more easily and with greater frequency.

Height is often thought to be a cause of back problems, especially in men. Many patients have been told that their backs are unstable, as they are so tall. This, they are told, is the cause of their pain. Similarly, several short, stocky men have been advised that their size makes them liable to back trouble.

In the course of my work, when I am called on to give evidence in court cases, they often involve the award of compensation for injury. In one extraordinary case, a six-foot, two-inch-tall woman had been in a car accident, and a doctor assessing her injuries said that fifty per cent of her back injuries were due to her height; this should be taken into account in reducing her claim, he said. When asked to comment, I pointed out that in my practice there was little difference in the incidence of back trouble at different heights and that I regarded her height as irrelevant.

Is there any connection between back pain and diet?

A common precipitating factor in the onset of a muscle cramp is a deficiency in calcium. The patient often suffers from cramps in the muscles of the calf or feet while resting, especially at night. They can be so bad that the sufferer needs to climb out of bed and walk about to relieve the pain. Cramps are generally worse at night because of the slowing of the arterial circulation. The lack of movement causes the muscles to have a fall in oxygen and an increase in waste products. This precipitates a cramp. Calcium can be given by injection or by mouth to prevent these cramps and bring long-lasting improvement. Some other trace elements such as magnesium can also reduce cramps.

Salt deficiency is a common cause of muscle cramp, although not often in the back. A deficiency is usually due to excessive sweating in very hot weather or during a high level of physical activity (the problem is known as Miner's Cramp). The salt level in the body falls to an unacceptably low level and the muscles go into a violent cramp. This may occur in any muscle and is made worse by exercise. A drink containing salt will usually bring instant relief.

If all the muscles in the body are in a near state of cramp due to any of these deficiencies then it follows that the muscles in the back may well become painful under conditions that would not normally affect them.

Could a food allergy lead to back pain?

Food allergies can be a precipitating factor in the onset of a muscle cramp and pain; while they are generally accepted as the cause of swollen joints, catarrh, fatigue and headaches, I have also noticed an occasional relationship between food and back pain. Indeed, I have referred several patients to food-allergy specialists to complement their treatment. Results have been most satisfactory.

The main allergic or sensitive condition that has an effect on the spine is a low-grade food allergy. We all know the acute type that occurs when you eat something like strawberries and shortly afterwards your face and other parts of the body become swollen and often covered in a rash. It is not this type of allergy but the lower grade allergy, or food intolerance as it is often called, that we are discussing here. Food intolerance is a term devised to avoid conflict between what medical experts deem criteria for an actual full-blown allergy, and just a food sensitivity. Common foods that are considered to cause 'intolerance' to many people are coffee, milk and white flour. Food intolerance can have the direct effect of causing a build-up of oedema in the group of muscles associated with the shoulder blade and joint, collectively known as the shoulder girdle and thereby lowering the threshold, making a painful cramp much more likely. Elimination of the offending food can have a marked effect on the onset of symptoms.

Food allergies are well covered in specialist books which I have recomended in the section on Further Reading (see page 242).

Do viral infections cause back pain?

Viral infections seem to be becoming more and more frequent and can sometimes be the cause of severe back pain. Many people, instead of catching a cold in the normal way, have a slight snuffle and then start to suffer pain in their backs. Often, they will show no obvious signs of a virus; usually they feel very tired or unwell and generally run down.

A viral infection gets into the bloodstream and travels all over the body. It settles in a muscle by entering the individual muscle fibres and multiplying in them. This causes inflammation of the muscle and can lead to pain.

A virus can attack the muscles in a normal back and be severe enough to immobilize the patient. People with bad backs, however, have an increased blood supply to the inflamed area and, as the infection is carried in the blood, the back receives a disproportionate amount of the infection. Once the infection has gone, then the back pain disappears and the back is usually left with no after-effects. Similarly, the increased level of activity caused by the infection on long-standing back trouble almost always reverts to the original level once the infection clears. Both the pain and the infection can be lessened with a short course of anti-inflammatory drugs.

Is my back pain due to the menopause?

Many women who are starting the menopause suffer aches and pains between the shoulders and in the lower part of the neck. This is caused by a deficiency of oestrins (female hormones) – normal at this time in a woman's reproductive cycle – which probably leads to an increase in the tissue fluids. Hormone Replacement Therapy (HRT), which replaces the body's lost hormones, can be most effective in ridding the patient of pain.

The other great advantage of HRT is that it acts to limit osteoporosis, or 'thinning of the bones'. It is most distressing to see women in their seventies and eighties with badly curved thoracic spines which are clearly very painful. Every so often I see an unfortunate patient who has a vertebra that has collapsed under the strain of its load. I believe that there are far too many older women with serious back problems due to decalcification of the vertebrae. Their pain could easily have been prevented with HRT in their earlier years.

It is hard to put the clock back to relieve such patients of their agony, but we can try to help others with HRT. Some women fear the risk of increased hormone-related cancers with HRT, but almost all the work in this country suggests there is no greater risk. It is also possible that a hormone-related cancer stimulated by HRT grows faster and so may be discovered earlier, before it has had any chance to spread.

In my experience HRT can not only drastically improve a patient's health, but also do a great deal to prevent the ravages of osteoporosis.

How is my back affected in pregnancy?

This is very complex question as there are several conflicting forces at work in your body at this very special time. As you will recall, the drug cortisone was discovered when medical researchers began looking into why women suffering from diseases such as rheumatoid arthritis suddenly felt the condition improve when they became pregnant. It was discovered that this was due to the fact that the suprarenal glands on top of the kidneys secreted a considerable increase of their product 'cortisone'. It is so called because it is the cortex – or outer layer – of the gland that secretes the substance.

This means that there is a powerful anti-inflammatory agent working throughout pregnancy which will tend to make a chronic (long-standing – *chronas* means time) back better to the point of being symptomless. After a while, however, the chemistry in the body changes in readiness to produce milk and this results in a relative deficiency in calcium.

Unfortunately, the lack of calcium makes the muscles more likely to go into cramp. Many an expectant mother suffers from cramps in her feet or calves at night which is a typical manifestation of a calcium shortage. The calcium deficiency affects the back muscles and makes them more sensitive so that back pain begins to be a possibility again.

Two more factors also tend to cause the back to be a problem in later months. The first is that the extra weight of the baby causes awkward stresses and an increased curve of the lumbar spine. This may lead to cramps of a very painful nature in the affected muscles. The situation is made worse by the fact that the ligaments of the pelvis begin to soften to allow expansion at the time of birth. The back muscles must therefore work harder to maintain posture. This again leads to an increased tendency to cramp.

To avoid these problems in pregnancy it is important to keep the calcium in the body at an adequate level by including calcium-rich foods (milk, cheese, sardines, broccoli) in your diet or taking it as a supplement if necessary. During pregnancy the body carries an increased quantity of fluid, thereby making oedema and circulation difficulties more likely. Exercises are also important to keep the circulation in the back muscles working as efficiently as possible.

If an expectant mother is known to have a back problem I find that it is best to give treatment after the second month of pregnancy as a precaution against trouble later on.

If the patient has a bad attack of pain in the last months of the pregnancy, treatment with surged faradism, ultrasonic waves and remobilization are safe (as long as the pregnancy is normal) and will almost always abolish the immediate pain. Ultrasonic waves are quite safe for the expectant mother. I usually suspend treatment at this point and suggest that it is resumed after the baby has been born.

Drugs should be avoided during pregnancy for although the anti-inflammatory drugs are not thought to cause problems they have not been proved to be safe.

Anthea, aged twenty-seven, came to see me when she was seven months' pregnant. She was in agony with lumbar (lower back) pain. She had suffered backache of a minor nature for some years. She said it was painful if she sat for too long or after carrying heavy shopping or standing over a sink or cooker.

Soon after she become pregnant her back felt altogether better and she had no pain at all. She was obviously

81

delighted and thought that her back problem was over. However, at about the sixth month she began to have cramps in her feet which would wake her up in the night. She often had to get out of bed to relieve them – and they were getting worse.

The day before I saw her she had been bending over to put a joint of lamb in the oven when she felt her back 'go'. The pain rapidly became agony and remained so until I saw her. I treated her with physical medicine which largely freed her of pain. The next morning she had a modest return of the pain so the following day I repeated the treatment. She had no further pain but still came to me five months later, as recommended, and was treated eight more times until all the spasm had gone.

Anthea has had no more backache for five years. She had another baby eighteen months after the first and was free of pain throughout the pregnancy.

4

BACK TO SPECIFICS

*Identifying pain associated
with your back*

> *There was a faith healer of Deal*
> *Who said 'Though the pain is not real*
> *If I sit on a pin*
> *And it punctures my skin*
> *I dislike the fancy I feel'.*

The previous two chapters have looked at the cause of back pain in a general way. We will now tackle the subject in more detail. In this chapter we study the individual structures of the back and the part they play in producing pain.

My father always held that 'nothing is as frightening as the unknown', pointing out that the best ghost stories did not give a detailed description of the ghost. They left it vague . . . to be filled in by the reader's own dark fears and anxieties. It is the same when patients are not given enough of the right kind of information about their complaints. That is why I feel it is so essential to lift the cloak of mystery from back pain and give sufferers an insight into their own particular problem. From the following summaries, you should be able to identify your specific problem from the different types of back pain discussed, and gain a better understanding of the cause of pain. At this point it is worth adding that I always encourage parents of children with back problems to include them in any discussion of the diagnosis and treatment.

Working in Partnership

Knowledge of your back should give you confidence to seek medical help and to keep pushing for treatment until you find relief from your back pain. I know from experience that a tremendous effort is often needed by patients to get doctors to recognize their back pain. Doctors are not always the most tolerant people. An embarrassing memory of my student days seems appropriate here. I was among a group of six new and nervous students gathered around an equally nervous and very frail middle-aged woman on our first day in hospital at the outpatient department. One of our number was singled out to question her. 'Well, have you found out what's wong with her?' asked the Great Physician. 'She has a painful back,' answered the student. This seemed to be the sum total of information that he had managed to extract. Suddenly, Sir lost patience. 'I am a very busy doctor,' he boomed loudly, just in front of the poor patient. 'She must not waste my time by coming to hospital complaining like this. All women have painful backs.'

For reasons which will be made clear throughout this book, back pain must be treated more seriously by doctors and sufferers. This chapter sets out to give sufferers a better understanding of their particular problem so they have the confidence to work in partnership with their doctor.

LUMBAR PAIN

This kind of pain varies greatly. It can be a slight ache or an extremely severe pain in the small of the back. The onset can be gradual over a period of days or quite sudden. It may even start instantaneously, accompanied by a loud click when the back feels as if something has 'gone out'. All these are probably variations of the same mechanism.

In previous chapters we have looked at the effect of a spasm on the muscles in the back. This symptomless spasm leads to a build-up of oedema in the tissues spaces, resulting in an increase in waste products and a lack of oxygen. When this condition reaches a critical state the muscle goes into cramp. Anything that either increases the demand for oxygen or nutrients, or further interferes with the action of the muscle pump helps take the condition of the muscle closer to a crisis level. Now, if a muscle is fairly near a cramp, then perhaps after a long car journey a few fibres of muscle may well go into cramp and you get a slight ache. You have the feeling that you want to wriggle your back a little to help it. This is nature's way of telling you to work the muscle pump and improve circulation.

If the muscles are nearer to a crisis, then many more fibres will go into cramp and the pain will be considerably worse. If all or nearly all the muscle goes into cramp then the pain is extremely severe and the patient may not be able to move. This same mechanism also accounts for pain higher up in the back.

What causes the 'click'?

There are several causes of the 'clicking' sound in joints. One of these is thought to be the bursting of a gas bubble when a joint is suddenly compressed. However, the 'click' that we are discussing here is when a muscle goes into cramp. This often happens when you are making a considerable muscular effort such as bending forward to lift something heavy. As you straighten, a muscle on the verge of a crisis may well go into a sudden acute cramp accompanied by a 'click'.

This 'click' is not, as many people imagine, a vertebra or disc being displaced. It is explained by the fact that the vertebrae, whether in an increased curve through bending, or rotated by a twisting movement, are off-centre to one another in relation to the bony projections.

As figure 4.1 shows, many of the muscles in the back are made up of a fleshy part which tapers into a thin wire-like tendon over much of its length. When a muscle suddenly goes into cramp, the spine is usually either bent forward or twisted at the time so one or more of these 'wires' may be directly on top of one of these projections. With the sudden tension of the cramp it may catch on the projection and flick on to the distant or wrong side of it with a distinct 'click'. Now while the muscle is stretched round this bone it is very difficult for it to come out of cramp. We have seen that muscles resent being stretched for extended periods of time and this applies even more when they are already in cramp. The agonizing pain can continue for a long time, usually somewhere between three days and three weeks until the muscle eventually becomes so fatigued that it relaxes and the tendon loosens. This slackened tendon can then pass back over the bone, allowing the muscle to shorten and to come out of the cramp.

A patient in extreme back pain is often put to bed until it subsides. Bed rest has been considered a 'cure' for so long it has become something of a habit with doctors. After a certain time in bed, a patient nearly always finds that a painful back feels better. The medical benefits of bed rest are rarely either advocated or disputed. The truth

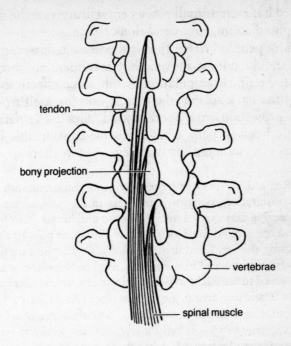

Figure 4.1 Some of the spinal muscles taper to thin wire-like tendons. When the muscle is in cramp the tendon can easily slip and hook on to the wrong side of the bony projection.

is, however, bed rest is of little positive help for a back-pain sufferer.

As we have just noted, the pain will indeed pass if you wait long enough for the muscle to weaken and relax, enabling it to free itself. After a certain time, your back will inevitably feel better, whether you are in bed or not. However, if a patient is encouraged to move about as much as possible this will speed up recovery of the muscle from the cramp because the muscle pump is improved. Obviously, the amount a patient can move may be very limited but even a small movement will activate the muscle pump and so improve conditions.

Many people believe that if a patient is in severe pain they should not be moved; but manipulation can often ease the pain. Manipulation at this stage effectively positions the back so that the muscle untraps itself from the bony projection with another loud 'click'. The patient is usually freed of pain, often for some considerable length of time, the moment the muscle is able to shorten.

Richard travelled all the way from Bournemouth for a consultation, lying on a mattress in the back of his estate car. He was carried into the house and he asked to be seen on the ground floor as he was in too much pain to attempt using the lift. I had just taken on a new assistant who was very experienced in the treatment of back problems and he agreed to see Richard whilst I finished with another patient.

When I returned, my new assistant had taken a history and done a quick examination. 'I'm afraid he is so bad he will have to stay in bed for two or three weeks to improve enough to be treated,' he told me. I was not so sure.

I explained to my assistant that if one could free the trapped muscle it would almost certainly come out of the cramp and revert to a symptomless state. Once I had tested Richard's back to see which way to manipulate him to untrap the muscle, I sat him on a stool and twisted him around to release the muscle. There was a loud 'click' and the severe pain stopped immediately. He was left with only a dull ache. After a course of treatment to relieve the basic spasm Richard has had no more attacks.

Why the relief is only temporary

I see a number of patients each year – like Fred, whose story is below – who have been having bouts of pain every few months. Each time they have been manipulated and relieved of pain. However, manipulation, while obviously being of great value in stopping pain, often only offers short-term relief. It does not help the underlying condition. The time may eventually come when the muscle is so sensitive that it goes into a cramp even though it is not stretched. When this happens, the muscle may not, of course, become trapped and so manipulation offers little help.

For about fourteen years, Fred, a thirty-eight-year-old packer, had been prone to lumbar pain. The attacks were usually fairly slight but on occasions – once or twice a year – they became very painful. Initially, he was put to bed for up to a fortnight and the pain eventually went each time but came back later. Then he had physiotherapy, which helped a little.

Fred thought he had found the answer to his problems when he found an osteopath who gave him immediate relief from his pain. He continued to go for osteopathy once or twice a year, whenever he had an attack, for ten years. Then, just five weeks before he came to see me, he said that for the first time he had got no relief from the manipulation.

The pain was so severe that he had tried heat, then bed rest and traction but it was to no avail. He was very troubled when he was told that he had to have an operation on his back but was advised to consult me first. When I saw him he was a little better but still in some pain and he was worried about the future. He added that he tired easily, had slight indigestion and became momentarily dizzy on suddenly standing up.

Fred stood with an increase in the curve of the lumbar spine and there was considerable spasm of the back muscles from the upper thoracic to the lower lumbar region. After eleven sessions of treatment, he had no further trouble with his back. Like so many of my patients, he was amazed and delighted at his fast and permanent recovery.

Other Common Back Problems

LOWER BACK PAIN

Trouble with the hip joints is a common reason for people complaining of lower back pain, usually on one side. Pain in the hip joint is generally felt in the buttock and sometimes slightly across the bottom of the back. There may also be pain in the groin. Pain may radiate down the back of the thigh to the knee and also from the groin obliquely down the front of the thigh to the inner side of the knee.

The hip joint is quite often overlooked as the cause. The diagnosis, however, is reasonably easy as movements that stretch the hip produce pain (see figure 1.12, on page 33). These movements include moving the leg out sideways, rotating the foot outwards or putting the knee across the other thigh.

You may remember from the earlier description that sacro-iliac joints are large flattish joints that form the part of the pelvis where the sacrum joins the pelvic basin (at the iliac bone). They are capable of little or no movement. A fairly severe blow may cause the ligaments which run across them to become stretched and many practitioners believe this allows one surface of the joint to slide on the other. As the surfaces are covered with irregular pits and humps (one side of the joint fitting exactly on to the other), it is thought that the joint may come to rest out of its true alignment.

The sacro-iliac joints are, in my experience, a much less common cause of pain in the lower back, except, perhaps, in pregnancy. Trouble in the sacro-iliac joints gives pain across the small of the back somewhat higher than the hip joint. The pain is usually on one side only. You feel pain if pressure is put directly on the joint or obliquely across the pelvis. This usually confirms the diagnosis.

SHOULDER AND NECK PAIN

- **Fibrositic pains between the shoulders** are cramps in the thoracic spinal muscles. There may also be cramps in the bundles of muscles that go under the shoulder blade from the spine to the shoulder. These cramps occur in muscles that are already in a spasm due to bruising of the facet joints in the area. This causes the pain to radiate from the spine outward underneath the shoulder blade to the actual joint.

  Many women who are starting the menopause experience pains or aches between the shoulders and in the lower part of the neck. This is due to a lack of oestrins during or after the menopause, which probably increases tissue fluids. As I mentioned in Chapter Three, Hormone Replacement Therapy (HRT) can be extremely beneficial. I have seen many patients whose pains have vanished and their health improved dramatically within days of starting the therapy.

- **A painful stiff neck** is almost always due to cramp in the muscles of the neck. Sometimes the big muscles going from the trunk to the skull, expecially the sterno-mastoid muscle which pulls the ear and head down and forward, join in with the cramp. This is not only painful but may also distort the head position.

- **A one-sided headache** may well be caused by a cramp in one of the small muscles just below the skull. The pain can be very intense and of a migraine type (see page 140). Pressure on the tender muscle often momentarily relieves pain.

REFERRED PAIN

Pains in the legs, arms, chest and other areas can be caused by back trouble. This is known as referred pain. The start of the problem is a nerve being irritated somewhere along its length. Far and away the most common cause of this is swelling of the facet joints. There are also a number of other causes, some of them common, such as an inflamed hip joint (which had inflamed a nerve running nearby), a bulging or ruptured disc, or tumours.

FACET JOINTS

As we have already seen, these joints can be bruised if the back is involved in a sharp jolt or jerking or twisting movement. Like any bruised joint, the facet joints can be swollen; normally, however, there is enough space around them to accommodate the swelling without causing a problem.

Sometimes, especially if the joint has become acutely inflamed, it swells into the neural canal so it can actually touch or squeeze the nerve (see figure 4.2). As a result, the patient feels referred pain in whatever part of the body the nerve supplies, most commonly the leg, quite often the arm and sometimes round the trunk.

The patient does not always suffer pain. Sometimes there are pins-and-needles or other sensations, and often there is numbness when the passage of impulses along the nerve from the area is blocked. Referred pain around the chest or in the abdomen is usually found in older patients, usually over the age of forty. If this is on the left side of the chest and/or down the left arm, it is very common for the pain to be mistaken for a coronary thrombosis. When the chest pain is referred from the back, an electro-cardiogram is, of course normal. Another distinction

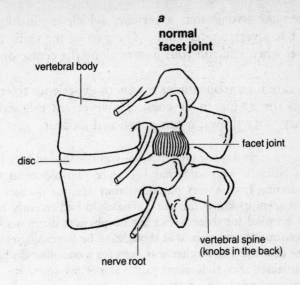

a
**normal
facet joint**

vertebral body

facet joint

disc

vertebral spine
(knobs in the back)

nerve root

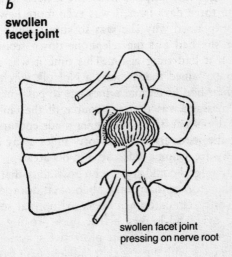

b
**swollen
facet joint**

swollen facet joint
pressing on nerve root

Figure 4.2 Diagram *a* illustrates a normal facet joint, *b* shows a swollen facet joint.

between the two is that a vertebra which is pinching a nerve has a very tender knob. (The part of the spine that you feel when you run your fingers along the centre of the back.)

It is rare for anyone under twenty to experience referred pain in the abdomen or chest. However, as this extraordinary story shows, it can occasionally occur.

In the early days of my practice I was telephoned by a lady in Norfolk who said that her seven-year-old child was suffering from a very painful tummy and the doctors did not seem to know the cause. The child had recently been in hospital for three weeks but no physical diagnosis had been made; the pain was thought to be psychological by the doctors. The mother was keen for a consultation but I explained that abdominal pain was not my speciality and recommended a paediatrician.

Imagine my surprise when she arrived in my consulting room three days later. I was even more bewildered when she explained why she was so sure I could help. Shortly after she had put the telephone down from our conversation it had rung again. This time it was a Mr Brown, who explained that he was a Norfolk witch and that his *familiar* had given him a message to pass on. He said that the message was that the source of the child's pain was actually in her back. The father made enquiries and found that the witch lived about forty miles away and was well known for helping sick cattle in his area.

Although I could still see no possibility that the pain was anything other than some abdominal disorder I examined the child. The abdomen appeared normal so I turned the child over and looked at her back. To my astonishment there was an area of acute protective spasm in the muscles of the back with a nerve that radiated pain from the associated vertebra to the exact spot in which the child was complaining of pain.

Treatment to the child's back rapidly relieved the pain

in her abdomen. I cannot pretend to say that I can explain this rather strange story but I just record it as a fact.

How can back trouble cause a painful calf or heel?

Referred pain is not easy to understand. To explain, let us compare the body to a hotel. Imagine you are in hotel-room number 512. As you press the bell to get room service an indicator board will flash room 512 and the maid will know where to go to get her instructions. A similar process occurs in the body. A nerve ending is represented by the bell push and the indicator board is in the brain. The brain therefore makes you aware that the origin of the sensation is at the actual point of stimulation; i.e., the heel.

Now let us suppose that some careless carpenter drives a nail through the insulation of the wire somewhere on its path from the bell push to the indicator board. The flasher would indicate that somebody was pushing the bell in 512 and the maid would not realize that the impulses were originating partway down the wire.

In the same way, as figure 4.3 shows, the brain thinks that the impulse originating from the neural canal in the spine is actually coming from the sensor at the nerve ending in the heel and so registers the pain as being there.

A nerve is like an electric cable with thousands of separate individual wires in the one sheath. When it is squeezed, hundreds of nerve fibres are usually involved, all sending their impulses to the brain – which misinterprets them as coming from their appropriate nerve ends. A patient may, for example, feel a sensation of pain from the thigh right down the leg to the foot, although, of course, the impulses actually originate only from the place where the nerve is being squeezed. Any pain, for whatever reason, in the sciatic nerve down the leg is called sciatica.

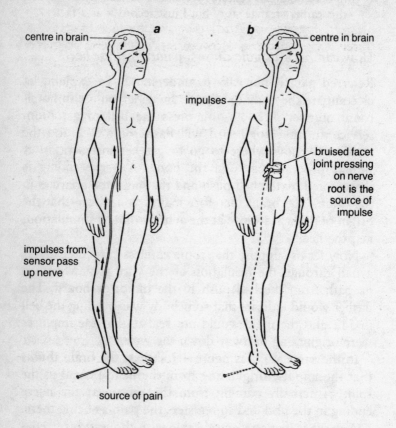

Figure 4.3 In diagram *a*, the source of pain in the foot (e.g., a pin prick) sends impulses from a sensor, up the nerve to the centre in the brain, where it is registered. In diagram *b*, however, where a facet joint has swollen to pinch the nerve root from the foot, the impulses pass along that same nerve, to the same part of the brain, which registers that the pain is in the foot.

THE INTERVERTEBRAL DISC

Although much-maligned, the disc, in my experience, rarely causes problems. However, it is still worth considering what can go wrong. As we have already seen, a disc is a flexible, tubular, fibrous box with a flat top and bottom welded on to the vertebrae above and below. It is full of an elastic jelly and behaves as if it was spongy rubber separating the two vertebrae. It has two functions, the obvious one of allowing movement in various planes between the two hard, flat vertebral faces (page 21) but also it is part of the mechanism for absorbing the shock of a blow to the spine (page 45). It is a very strong structure and, in my view, is seldom damaged.

What can go wrong with a disc?

There are three possible things that can go wrong with a disc.

- Firstly, the disc can be compressed as muscles in spasm put pressure on the adjacent vertebrae. If you imagine sitting on two tins with thick spongy rubber between, it is clear that under this pressure a disc may well bulge. If it bulges into the neural canal it may touch the nerve (see figure 4.4 diagram *b*). This will not cause pain from the disc itself but, as we have seen in the previous section, in the origin of the nerve. Occasionally the local cramp of the muscles is felt as back pain but the intense referred pain is so overwhelming that this is often hardly noticeable.

  This condition is fairly easily corrected by treatment that relaxes the spasm of the muscles. This takes the pressure off the disc and allows it to return to a normal shape, thus relieving the pressure on the nerve. The disc

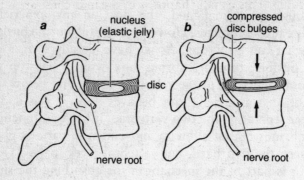

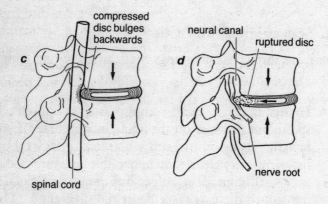

Figure 4.4 Intervertebral disc problems. Diagram *a* indicates a normal, healthy disc. Diagram *b* shows the disc compressed by a muscle spasm, bulging out and touching the nerve root. Diagram *c* shows the same thing, but bulging backwards to the spinal cord. Diagram *d*, less frequent, is the result of a ruptured disc. Note how the contents of the disc (nucleus) have escaped, compressing the nerve root.

may also bulge directly backwards touching the spinal column. This usually happens in the mid-chest area. (See figure 4.4, diagram *c*).

The spinal cord is very large in diameter and occupies most of the space available in the canal. As a result, if a disc that is being compressed by the spasm bulges backwards it can touch the spinal cord, resulting in impulses being sent up to the brain from the affected area. This usually causes pain – not where the disc is, but at the very base of the spine, and this usually radiates into one thigh. When severe, the pain can be in the back, some way down one leg, and in the other buttock.

• The second and more serious cause of pain from a disc is when as a result of prolonged pressure from the muscle spasm, the fibrous wall of the disc ruptures and the jelly pours out (see figure 4.4, diagram *d*). This tends to stretch the nearby nerve passing through the canal. The nerve continues to be stretched as the jelly increases in density and begins to solidify after it has been out of the disc for a while. Although there is often little or no pain locally, the inflamed nerve sends impulses to the brain which again misinterprets them as coming from the beginning of the nerve.

• Thirdly, and this is very rare indeed, the fibrous wall of the disc could be ruptured by an acute injury, such as a fall from a height, and the result is the same as in the second group.

The vast majority of patients feel pain in the sciatic nerve down the leg; however it is also possible to feel pain in the foot, arm, round the body or in the chest according to the positioning of the disc and nerve. If a disc has ruptured then the pain is severe and relentless. However, in my experience a disc lesion is comparatively rare.

Looking at the underlying problem

Of the several hundred back-pain sufferers whom I see each year, on average only one has a ruptured disc. I have always felt that the disc is exaggerated as a cause of back problems. Too much research is devoted to the various attributes of the disc and not enough to what may actually be causing the problem.

You could say that it is rather like having a bus shelter that is continually being hit by a bus. Sophisticated research is carried out to find the best materials to make a bus shelter strong enough to minimize damage and endless statistics are compiled on the design of the shelter, but all the time a simple tightening of a loose nut on the steering of the bus could solve the problem completely.

Many of the problems of the back do not cause symptoms that are directly associated with it. Although a patient may not feel pain in the back itself, the underlying problem in the spinal column can still affect nearby structures and systems and cause serious problems in other parts of the body. This often results in a number of well-known disorders not usually associated with the back, and also a new disease. These will be considered in the next three chapters.

5

BACK TO FRONT

Your back problem
and a new disease

Patient: 'I hope you will find that I am ill.'
Doctor: 'What do you want to be ill for?'
Patient: 'I would hate to be well and feel as I do.'

Patients often come to me saying they feel unwell, but no one seems to be able to pinpoint the real cause. Tiredness, depression, indigestion, dizzy spells and headaches, together with a general feeling of being 'not quite right' are common symptoms. Many of these people have been given treatment for one or more of the symptoms individually but often they say that it has had no lasting effect.

Given these symptoms, a full investigation is obviously necessary; a very important step is always to examine the patient's back. It is my firm belief that – if none of the better known causes have been found – the back is usually the source of the problem. I find that once the back is treated then the illness also clears up. Often the back is symptomless; sometimes it is painful. In either case, it is rarely associated with the illness and so patients, where possible, receive only symptomatic treatment, which does nothing to cure the overall trouble. It is a sad fact that tens of thousands of people are suffering with little hope of finding an answer to their problems.

I would like to illustrate this with the story of a prominent businessman who came to see me some years ago. I diagnosed the cause of his symptoms as silent back trouble and after several treatment sessions he was back on top form.

Lord D., a prominent businessman and well-known workaholic, complained that recently he had started to feel excessively tired and, at times, very depressed. He also had difficulty in concentrating and was beginning to fight shy of anything that was likely to put him under pressure.

He told me that he had been to see his GP and asked to be sent to a top consulting physician to find out what was wrong. He was put in a nursing home for three weeks and all his body fluids were analysed; he was X-rayed and scopes were put in through every orifice possible.

Eventually, Lord D. found himself sitting in front of the physician who had a pile of test results, inches high, on his desk. He explained that the physician tapped his knees and ankles and listened to his chest then said, 'I am very happy to tell you that there is absolutely nothing wrong with you at all.' Well aware that Lord D.'s name was often in the paper connected with takeover bids, he added, 'When did you last take a holiday?'

Lord D. confessed that it was probably five or six years since he had really had a break. Convinced by the doctor that a lack of holiday was the cause of the problem, Lord D. packed his bags and spent three months on a restful holiday in the South of France.

The holiday did little to relieve the symptoms and so Lord D. asked to be referred to another consultant. The consultant looked through the large pile of tests that had been done, tapped his knees and ankles and listened to his chest and said there was absolutely nothing wrong. He continued by asking, 'What have you been doing with yourself recently?' When Lord D. told him that he had been in the South of France for three months the immediate reply was, 'Well, all that's wrong with you is that you need a jolly good job of work.'

In many instances these doctors may have been right to recommend a change in routine to help relieve these mysterious ailments. However, there are also many people like Lord D. for whom an examination of the back provides the necessary clues to the problem. Lord D. was suffering from a disease which is very common and fortunately is usually easy to correct. Before we look at this disease in more detail it is important that you understand the role tissue fluids play in the body as this is crucial to understanding the problem.

EFFECTS OF A POOR MUSCLE PUMP

We have discussed how a damaged or bruised facet joint causes a protective spasm of the muscles across it. This spasm, because of the pressure it exerts on the joint, maintains the bruising, thus the problem in the back is self-perpetuating. Under these conditions there may well eventually be symptoms in the back itself, usually pain.

The problem, however, may spread further in the body than the spine and cause a number of other ailments. The blame for this lies with the diminished activity of the muscle pump when the muscle is in spasm.

As noted in Chapter One, when a muscle contracts it compresses not only its own tissues but also the adjacent tissues. This action squeezes fluid and blood out of the tissues. Apart from those areas affected by gravity, this is the body's main mechanism for taking the blood from the tissues and returning it to the heart. If spasm causes the muscle pump to work poorly then this pumping action is slowed down.

Earlier, we looked at the effect of this poor pumping on the tissues of the back muscles. Now let us study how it affects the adjacent tissues. One of the most important of these is the sympathetic nerve chain which lies close to the spinal muscles in the lower neck and upper thoracic part of the spine. It is one of three separate but inter-dependent nerve systems present in the body. These are:

1. **The central nervous system.** This is the most important nerve system. It is dominated by the brain and also includes all the ordinary sensory and motor nerves that run all over the body. The central nervous system controls all voluntary actions and perceives all conscious sensations such as vision, taste and smell, hearing, skin sensations, muscle, joint and tendon status, and the pain of internal malfunctions such as an injury or appendicitis. See figure 5.1, for the position of this system in the body.

2. **The sympathetic nervous system.** This chain of nerve centres is connected by nerves to each other, to the spinal nerves and to virtually every part of the body. It influences the running of the entire body machine and monitors and controls a vast number of parameters such as blood pressure, blood chemistry and repair. It is also responsible for the body's built-in response in emergency situations.

Why 'sympathetic'? Well, this is actually rather an unfortunate name for this system. It is probably more related to the French word *sympathique*, as it was noticed that this system caused an increased heart beat in an emotional situation. However, in reality, this is only because it is part of the adrenalin mechanism which is designed to put the body into a state of efficiency in an emergency. This has been fully discussed in Chapter Three.

In primitive conditions, this kind of emergency would be a purely physical one. The sympathetic nervous system

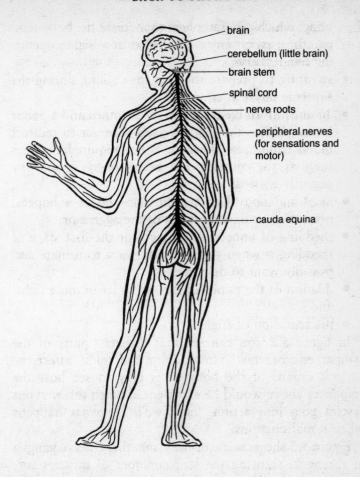
brain

cerebellum (little brain)

brain stem

spinal cord

nerve roots

peripheral nerves
(for sensations and
motor)

cauda equina

Figure 5.1 The central nervous system, which runs throughout the whole body.

prepares the body for instant and intense action. As it does so, the person will experience:

- a rise in pulse and blood pressure;
- small contractions of a number of muscles, or trem-

bling, which generates heat to increase the body temperature; everything works better at a higher operating temperature;

- sweating to prepare the skin for cooling during the supreme physical effort;
- an uncomfortable feeling in the stomach and a pallor in the skin as the blood vessels contract to redirect blood from areas where it is not required to areas such as the muscles and brain where it may be urgently needed;
- head and body hair standing on end as a hopeful protection against the teeth of the aggressor;
- shedding of unnecessary weight or the first stage of shedding it when you feel sick, want to urinate and possibly want to defecate;
- dilation of the pupils of the eye to let in more light; and
- the sensation of fright.

In figure 5.2 you can see that different parts of the sympathetic nervous system, along the spine, affect the various organs of the body. It is easy to see how the responses above would be experienced when this nervous system goes into action. Later we'll see what happens when it malfunctions.

Figure 5.3 shows some of the sympathetic nerve ganglia in the neck, showing the large number of muscles surrounding these. It is clear how tensing of these muscles would affect those ganglia.

3. **The parasympathetic nervous system.** Also known as the vegative system, this mainly controls the digestive tract, and its stimulation causes secretion of digestive juices and the churning movement of the stomach and bowel after food. It also opposes and balances the sympathetic nervous system throughout most of the

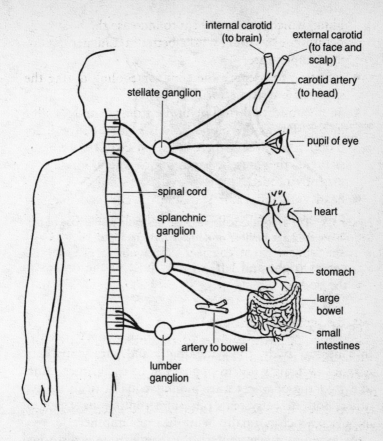

Figure 5.2 The sympathetic nervous system. The nerve centres (ganglia) are linked to specific organs in the body, and these are the organs which are adversely affected when the sympathetic nervous system is under pressure.

body. It consists of a nerve centre in the brain and a long nerve which wanders all over the body and is called the 'vagus', meaning wandering. This system is basically the opposite of the sympathetic nervous system. As you can see from figure 5.4, the vagus

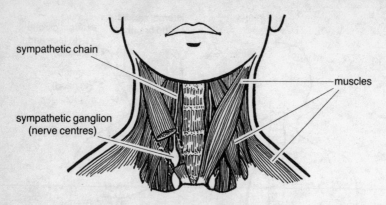

Figure 5.3 The sympathetic nerve chain lies close to the base of the neck. Note the large number of muscles surrounding it.

nerves (right and left) supply most of the organs in the body.

Tug-of-war situation

In a healthy body, the sympathetic and parasympathetic nervous systems work in opposition to each other rather like two tug-of-war teams pulling equally against each other. Both nerve systems put out a continuous stream of impulses which normally neutralize one another.

As in a tug-of-war contest, this equilibrium is disturbed when the output of one nerve system is increased or decreased. If, for example, something were to diminish the effect of the sympathetic nervous system, then the normal pull of the parasympathetic previously neutralized would now make it active. As the sympathetic nerve system slows down, the parasympathetic becomes dominant.

Under normal conditions, if one nerve system is stimulated then the other almost switches off. When, for example, the sympathetic system is activated through fear, the parasympathetic has little output so that energy is

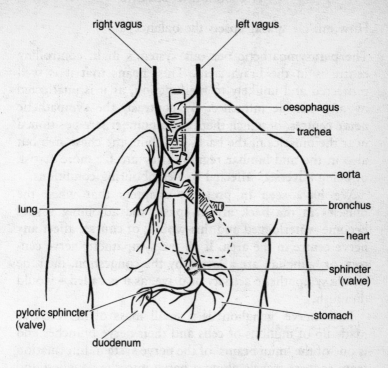

Figure 5.4 The vagus nerve (right and left) runs throughout the body, parallel to the sympathetic nervous system. It is the mainstay of the parasympathetic nervous system and we can blame the vagus nerve for excessive fatigue.

not wasted during the crisis by, say, the continuation of digestion. If the crisis lasts only a few minutes, as it would have done in primitive times, then this does not lead to problems. However, if anything causes a prolonged imbalance, this can have far-reaching effects on the normal functioning of the body.

How muscle spasm upsets the balance

The parasympathetic nervous system's main controlling centre is in the brain stem. This means that it is well protected and unlikely to malfunction, as it is unaffected by any outside influence. By contrast, the sympathetic nerve centres, of which there are a number, are positioned near the muscles of the back, mainly in the chest area but also in the mid-lumbar region. They are far more at risk of being adversely affected by neighbouring conditions.

We have seen in previous chapters that when the muscles in the back are in spasm the adjoining tissues become waterlogged and this would, of course, affect any nerve centre in the area. If all the sympathetic nerve centres, or 'ganglia', are affected by the congestion, then the whole sympathetic activity or drive, as it is called – would diminish.

Each nerve 'ganglion' is a small mass of nerve tissue made up of millions of cells and their nerve branches and is one of the 'mini brains' of the nerve system. Information from sensors travels along a nerve into the ganglion and arrives at a gap between that nerve and another nerve cell. Exactly as in a computer, this information is passed to, or blocked from, the next nerve; but by chemicals generated in the gap by other nerves which control the transmission. The effect of a large chain of such reactions results in appropriate correcting messages being sent to the tissues concerned. This may well also be affected by information from other sources. Look at figure 5.2 to see how each of the ganglia of the sympathetic nervous system supplies various parts of the body. The proper monitoring of the impulses by this chemical control is therefore easily upset by excessive fluid in the ganglion.

In a situation when the sympathetic activity has been slowed down, it follows then that the vagus (or wandering) nerve supplying the same area, being relatively unopposed, would have excessive activity. A patient would show symptoms both of a low sympathetic drive and also of extra activity of the vagus (see page 108).

This combination of symptoms and signs results in a new syndrome which I have named 'HypoSympathetic Tone', or HST for short. 'Hypo' means low or below normal. Although previously unrecognized, this disease seems to affect a large number of people.

One the most dominant symptoms of HST is that the patient tires easily. This is especially noticeable if there is no challenge. Pressure situations such as decisions at work raise the sympathetic drive and help to override the tiredness. However, once the pressue is off then the patient usually flakes out.

Here's an example of the condition manifesting itself in someone quite young.

Jonathan was only sixteen when he came to see me. Two years previously he had felt extremely tired for three months. Despite intensive investigations no reason was found and it was put down to a poor diet and pressure at school. He improved spontaneously and went back to his normal life. But six months before I saw him he suddenly became very tired again for no apparent reason. He said he felt like going to bed nearly all the time. He started to have momentary dizzy or faint feelings if he stood suddenly. He was also extremely tense and had moments when he felt depressed.

As I suspected, he told me that he had fallen off a horse six years previously and had landed on the back of his shoulders. When I examined him there was a spasm of the spinal muscles caused by the old injury to his thoracic spine, which had bruised the facet joints. There was a spasm of the spinal muscles from the neck to the low thoracic region and an increase in the thoracic curve. The spasm of the muscles had caused oedema in the area and this had depressed the sympathetic nervous system, causing tiredness. Dizziness was caused by ensuing momentary falls in blood pressure. I treated him with physiotherapy and manipulation of his thoracic spine but Jonathan's problem took a long time to cure. Although he felt vastly better after six visits he kept relapsing a little and needed more treatment. Finally, after twenty-eight visits over one and a half years he was well and stayed well.

A New Disease

HST affects a large number of people and can, when severe, cause considerable distress and incapacity. Although the disease is unrecognized at present, it is readily diagnosed and can be successfully treated. The symptoms fall into four main groups:

- effects of the low sympathetic drive;
- effects of parasympathetic over-activity;
- compensatory reactions of the brain; and
- thoracic and lower neck trouble.

Let us look at each of these symptom groups in more detail.

EFFECTS OF THE LOW SYMPATHETIC DRIVE

Extreme tiredness is usually the first and only symptom for several years. After a time, patients feel not only tired but also unwell. Sometimes they can become seriously ill.

- **Tiredness** caused by the low sympathetic drive has certain distinct characteristics. It seems to peak at around three or four in the afternoon after which the patient usually perks up again. Sufferers also tend to flake out when they arrive home from work but can be revived quickly by a short rest. Indeed, it seems that excessive tiredness at any time of the day can be relieved by a rest or sleep of as little as five or ten minutes.

Restful holidays are often recommended to sufferers but they are not a great success for anyone with HST. As we have already seen, the sympathetic nervous system needs a challenge to maintain a reasonable level of drive and so a restful holiday is seldom helpful. Even if it is, the patient seems to go right back to square one in a few weeks after returning and might just as well not have gone away.

- **Low blood sugar** is another symptom of a low sympathetic drive. Patients may have sudden attacks of low blood sugar which makes them feel weak and cold – sometimes with a clammy sweat. They may also experience a sense of unease, even a feeling of impending doom.
- **Low blood pressure** is also a common sign. In most cases it is very much at the lower end of what is usually regarded as normal. Patients often say their blood pressure has been rather low for a number of years but they were not aware that it was a problem. Common effects of low blood pressure are dizzy spells and a faint feeling when you stand up suddenly, especially after having been lying down.

If the patient is in late middle age and has had the problem for many years, the blood pressure often begins to rise suddenly, and tends to become excessively high. It may need treatment to lower it to within normal limits.

EFFECTS OF PARASYMPATHETIC OVER-ACTIVITY

- **Indigestion** of some form is a very common symptom. The high level of acid inflames the stomach lining making it extremely sensitive. This may show itself in a fairly mild way. Often patients say that they cannot stop nibbling. This is nature's way of mopping up the excess acid in the stomach caused by the activity of the parasympathetic nervous system.

Some patients lose their appetite as the stomach resents food being put into it. They may also complain of frequent belching. This is actually subconscious swallowing of air in an effort to separate the sensitive walls of the stomach. The patient can be very difficult to persuade that they are not in fact bringing the air up. If the condition gets even worse then there may be indigestion with symptoms of a leaden weight feeling or pain in the stomach. In extreme circumstances, a gastric or duodenal (intestinal) ulcer may result.

- **Allergic reaction** may occur as the inflamed stomach becomes unusually sensitive to irritating foods. If this happens, it will sometimes activate the early warning system in the body which enables tissues to recognize a minute trace of a substance that has caused trouble previously.

It is rather like an army that has on a number of occasions suffered a full-scale assault by the enemy, preceded by the sighting of a few patrols. So one day when a patrol wearing the recognizable uniform of the aggressor army shows itself, an immediate full-scale mobilization will take place, even though the enemy army is on this occasion actually not present. In the same way, the body will react in a normal manner to this known irritant, but at a level that is excessive and totally out of proportion to the very small amount of it present.

These allergies usually regress as the stomach improves with treatment to the protective spasm in the back muscles. Occasionally, however, they do need treating in their own right.

COMPENSATORY REACTIONS OF THE BRAIN

- **Tension** is often a dominant symptom of HST. To explain the reason for this I would like to compare the low sympathetic drive to having a low voltage in an all-electric house. You have no idea that the voltage is low but you do notice that the lights are a bit dim and that the cooker does not get as hot as it used to. The washing machine is not working well, nor is the television, hi-fi system or any of the other electrical appliances. You call in specialists for each individual appliance to test them but they cannot find anything wrong.

In the same way, doctors trying to diagnose someone with HST may find that each individual system appears to be normal. The filaments in the light bulbs are intact and of the correct resistance. The cooker heater elements are normal and the thermostats are all in working order. Naturally, you are left wondering whether you are imagining things. However, if the specialists had looked beyond the working of the applicances to the voltage coming into the house they would have found the reason for the inefficiency.

Fortunately, the body has sensors which alert the brain to the fact that the sympathetic drive is low. Just like the house owner who is tired of the poor-working electric appliances, so the brain gets fed up with the unsatisfactory

115

running conditions in the body and resolves to do something to correct things.

As we have already seen, when someone has had a shock the anxiety/fright centre stimulates the sympathetic nerve centres (ganglia). When the sympathetic nervous system is flagging, the brain tries to perk it up by simulating an anxiety and thus activating the anxiety/fright centre. This results in the patient becoming very tensed up. Most people think that being tensed up causes stomach and other problems when, in fact, they are both the result of the same illness.

- **Depression** has many causes, but can also be one of the symptoms of HST. Sadly, if the patient has no apparent worries, or has a depressive personality, then this tensed-up state can lead to attacks of depression which may be serious enough to consult a psychiatrist.

A tense state of mind is a mild version of fright, however, the body reacts with a physical reaction designed for a crisis in the jungle. Among the effects of this emergency response, the muscles of the shoulder girdle and thoracic spine tense up ready for the impending battle. This further interferes with the muscle pump and so further aggravates the malfunction of the sympathetic nerve centres (see page 110). Under these conditions a patient often feels even more tensed up and a limited vicious circle is set up.

- **Inability to cope with a change in routine** is another classic symptom. Patients find it hard to cope with events out of their normal range of life. This is because the subconscious brain, realizing that the defence mechanism is not working properly, tries to stop you going out of the cave. It suspects that if you were to meet a wild animal you might not – without the benefit of a sympathetic boost – be able to cope with it. Even an invitation to be sociable with friends could seem too daunting and all sorts of excuses are conjured up in an attempt to avoid something that appears to the subconscious to be an impending confrontation.

In reality, the best possible thing for the patient would be to go to the social event. As soon as they arrived they'd see there was no danger and could enjoy themselves.

Some while ago Stephen was practically frog-marched in for a consultation by two concerned friends. Ten years previously he had started to feel rather tired and although he was normally very sociable, he had gradually become more and more reluctant to go out to dinner or to other events. As time passed a modest reluctance turned into a marked liability and he became quite anti-social.

Stephen's friends became alarmed when he started taking mornings and then days off work because he felt too tired or said that he could not cope with events at the time. Before long, it got so bad that he rarely left his home. The final straw for his friends was when he started asking for food to be sent up to his room as he found it altogether too much to go downstairs to eat.

Stephen had seen a pyschiatrist a few years before who said that he was somewhat depressed and needed a holiday. The holiday had done him no good and the feeling of inertia had gradually increased. When I asked him about any back trouble he seemed puzzled but revealed that he had had intermittent neck trouble and pains between his shoulders for many years. It transpired that about fifteen years before he had been involved in a car accident, when he had suffered a whiplash injury.

On examination, it was clear that his sympathetic nerve

centres had been involved when the facet joints were bruised by the injury and had become waterlogged. The brain had over-reacted in its endeavour to increase the sympathetic drive. Once the back was treated he started to feel his old self again.

SYMPTOMS FROM THORACIC AND LOWER NECK TROUBLE

We have already seen how back trouble in the thoracic and lower neck areas of the spine can depress the activity of the sympathetic nerve ganglia, which lie close to the affected muscles. It follows then that a symptom of HST may be pain in these parts. Patients often complain of fibrositic (inflammation of the fibrous tissue of the muscle sheaths), or non-arthritic pain between the shoulders and/or base of the neck. On examination there is usually considerable spasm of the paravertebral muscles in the area.

Is There a Cure for HST?

Through recognizing and understanding the underlying problem causing HST, I have formulated a successful treatment for the disease. This treatment will be covered in detail in the final chapter of the book. By healing the trouble causing the imbalance between the sympathetic and parasympathetic nervous systems, the harmony between the two is restored and the various symptoms disappear. Thankfully, the treatment has restored the good health of the majority of sufferers. On page 246, there is a letter from one such sufferer.

Other Back-related Diseases

The disease of HypoSympathetic Tone (HST) involves the whole sympathetic system. Although it is common it is far more common to have only one or two centres affected by the back trouble. Most of the problems mentioned in low sympathetic drive syndrome occur on their own and are, of course, recognized as separate diseases such as migraine and indigestion. The way these problems have cleared up when the associated part of the back has been put right leads me to believe that a number of people who suffer from these problems have a partial sympathetic imbalance associated with back trouble as their primary problem. This will be discussed in detail in Chapter Seven.

However, before looking at these complaints I would like to discuss a mysterious disease, commonly known as ME or Chronic Fatigue Syndrome, that affects a great number of people. You may be asking what ME has to do with back pain but in the next chapter I shall show how the symptoms fit my theory of back problems and their related illnesses and why many patients respond so well to the appropriate treatment. By relieving sufferers of their underlying back trouble, I have helped them considerably and in many cases provided complete relief.

6

YOUR BACK AND ME

*Why ME or Chronic Fatigue
Syndrome is not such a
mysterious disease*

The disease known as ME has been given a variety of names including Icelandic Disease – the country where it was originally diagnosed – and the Royal Free disease, named after the hospital where the first recognized out-break occurred in Britain. Post-Viral Syndrome is another commonly used title for the disease. It has been given another name, and one which I prefer: Chronic Fatigue Syndrome. As a 'syndrome' it also covers those cases that are not obviously associated with an infection.

The name Myalgic Encephalomyelitis (ME) seems less satisfactory to me. My reasons will become clear throughout this chapter. Firstly, I doubt whether the encephalon – another name for the brain – is often, if ever, involved in the disease except in cases of extreme severity. Secondly, myalgia (meaning a number of painful muscles) is usually ascertained by an ESR test (Erythrocyte Sedimentation Rate), which measures the settling proper-ties of red cells in blood. This is calculated by placing blood in a vertical tube and observing the quantity that settle in the bottom of the tube after an hour. Curiously this is a very sensitive measure of the degree of activity of the defence mechanism when the body is responding to either an inflammatory or an infectious disease. A raised test result under these conditions usually indicates Polymyalgia. In patients suffering from ME the ESR remains normal as do most other tests.

CLARIFYING THE CONFUSION

'Encaphalon' means 'the brain', and 'Myelos' is the Greek for 'marrow'. The spinal cord was once thought to be marrow, in the centre of the bones, so the word now also means 'to do with the spinal cord'. 'Itis' does of course mean 'inflammation of'. Therefore, Encephalomyelitis is an inflammation of the brain and spinal cord, and it causes a number of the symptoms found in ME. These include tiredness, depression, muscle weakness and pain, and sensory symptoms such as pins and needles. There is, however, a much more simple alternative explanation for these symptoms, which I will discuss later in this chapter.

Myalgic Encephalomyelitis can occur with a virulent (very severe) attack of a number of common virus infections. Most sufferers who have this particular problem are treated in specialized units; this grave condition is quite rare.

The disease is poorly understood by many people. Indeed, some doctors believe it is simply a figment of the imagination. Such confusion means that people suffering from other somewhat similar diseases are classed as ME or Chronic Fatigue Syndrome patients and this makes it difficult to integrate the signs and symptoms into a single disease.

To shed some light on this difficult problem, let us look more closely at the particular disease that I prefer to call Chronic Fatigue Syndrome. Many of the symptoms were apparent in a fifty-five-year-old bank manager who came to see me recently.

Joe had been feeling very slightly off-colour for several

years but he put it down to the onset of old age. Five years before he had suffered an attack of influenza and was left feeling very tired and depressed for several weeks. After about six months he felt flu-like symptoms once more and this was followed by both depression and, more distressing, a feeling of complete exhaustion. He had only to do the slightest thing such as get up and walk in the garden and he felt completely knocked out and had to go to bed for at least twenty-four hours.

Joe had further slight flu-like attacks every few months for about a year. Just as he was starting to feel better in himself, he would be hit by the symptoms again. He started to feel pains in his legs, especially the left, and they became very heavy. He also had aches in his neck and shoulders and suffered mild indigestion. A more constant and, to Joe, more worrying symptom was a woolly feeling in his head, lack of concentration and an obvious slowness of thought.

When Joe came to see me he was so low that he had been unable to work for about two and a half years. However, he said he was feeling some improvement after following a suitable diet and taking Vitamin B supplements.

When I examined him I found the typical results of a previous injury to his thoracic spine, i.e., intense spasm of the muscles from the neck to the lower thoracic part of the back.

These are by no means all the possible symptoms of the Chronic Fatigue Syndrome but I have chosen Joe as a good representative case. After treatment, which I shall describe in the last chapter, Joe's condition rapidly improved and he was soon back to full-time work.

What Is the Cause?

Several different medical specialists are researching the cause and treatment of Chronic Fatigue Syndrome. Their findings are varied and tend to be linked with their own particular speciality. Thus, a virologist (a bacteriologist who specializes in viral diseases) may believe it to be caused by an entero virus (which mainly infects the bowel, for example coxsakie) or other virus, whereas the food allergy expert would demonstrate the improvement obtained by treating food allergies. Curiously, hand-in-hand with this goes a candida infestation, especially of the bowel, which we will discuss later in this chapter. Inevitably, there are also those who believe it to be a psychological complaint, especially because the results of clinical tests are usually normal. Others do not believe that, as an illness, it exists at all.

I have been consulted by a number of people suffering from this disease and now believe it to be the result of an almost complete shutdown of the sympathetic nervous system. This is caused by two separate problems which, put together, give the picture of the Chronic Fatigue Syndrome. The underlying problem is the wide-reaching effects of a severe injury to the chest area of the spine as in Joe's case. As we have seen, such an injury can result in a low sympathetic drive with associated complaints. The second problem arises when a patient already suffering from a low sympathetic drive is affected by an attack of influenza or similar acute infectious disease which further upsets the sympathetic chain and lowers the body's resistance to infection.

If a person has had an injury to the chest area of the spine as a result of, say, slipping and falling over backwards, there will be a protective spasm of the paravertebral muscles in this area. This will interfere with the normal function of the muscle pump and lead to a build-up of oedema both in the muscles themselves and also in the adjoining tissues.

The body's own sewage farm

As we have already discussed, the sympathetic nerve centres may be affected by the build-up of oedema leading to many of the symptoms of low sympathetic drive. Unfortunately, the sympathetic nervous system is not the only system that may be involved. Intermingled with the nerve centres are numerous lymph nodes. These are part of the lymphatic system, a special mechanism for dealing with an infection, damage or foreign bodies in the tissue spaces.

In order to get a good picture of the role of the lymph nodes it may help to look back to some of the points raised in Chapter One concerning the circulation of the blood. We saw that when the blood reaches the capillaries, fluid diffuses from the blood into the tissue spaces taking in supplies and oxygen. It then diffuses back into the other end of the capillaries carrying with it carbon dioxide and waste products. The blood system is able to a great extent to keep out undesirable foreign bodies such as bacteria, viruses, white cells that have engulfed some invader, and the broken-down remains of debris.

During the transfer there is no direct connection between the blood vessels and the tissue spaces, so clearly some mechanism for the removal and disposal of foreign bodies is needed. This is where the lymphatic system comes in (see figure 6.1). As the lymphatic ducts are in direct communication with the tissue spaces they act as the sewers of the body and make it possible for these small particles to be removed. The moment any infection gets into the tissue spaces the bacteria and viruses and any foreign bodies are swept up by the tissue fluids into the lymph ducts where they become lymph. The driving force is a massive increase in the blood supply which is part of the body's response to the infection and, of course, the muscle pump.

124

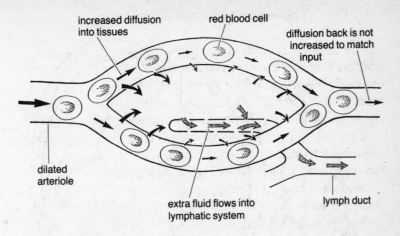

Figure 6.1 When inflamed (by bruise or infection) the arteriole dilates, increasing the blood flow into the capillary, and thus into the tissue spaces. Some of this tissue fluid goes into the lymphatic system, taking with it bacteria, minute foreign bodies and white blood cells.

The bacteria and viruses pass up the ducts either independently or, after being engulfed, in the white cell soldiers of the body. Either way, they are accompanied by cells, other debris and undesirable chemicals present in the tissue spaces. After being processed the lymph passes into the final lymph ducts and these join into the huge veins at the top of the chest. Lymph nodes can be compared to a sewage farm; the lymph node filters and detoxifies the lymph as it passes through.

As figure 6.2 shows, there are chains of lymph nodes which ensure that the lymph is reasonably pure by the time it is returned to the bloodstream. This is important because the arterial system has little power to deal with such problems. At the same time, a special mechanism produces antibodies that are lethal to particular organisms. Each antibody works against one type of bacterium

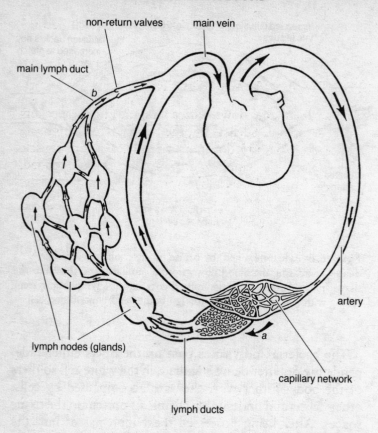

Figure 6.2 The lymphatic system runs parallel to the circulatory system. At point *a*, the tissue fluids, containing waste, bacteria and minute solids, pass into the lymph, where they are cleaned. At point *b*, the main lymph duct, cleaned fluid and antibodies are returned to the vein, and the circulatory system.

only so that the body has many antibodies to cover a wide range of bacteria and viruses that may invade the body.

Now, if the muscle pump is not working properly and there is a build-up of oedema in the local tissues, then these lymph nodes, or filters, will also be affected. If they

126

too are blown out with fluid then they may well become less efficient.

EFFECTS OF A VIRAL INFECTION

When a patient goes down with a viral infection, especially a fairly severe one such as flu, the lymphatic system has a great deal of work to do. If, as a result of a poor muscle pump action, the lymph nodes are already over-loaded, they will become even more water-logged than before. This, of course, makes it difficult for the patient to throw off the current infection and also lowers the body's resistance to any future infections. Thus, we have the usual history of an acute flu-like infection starting the illness off and then the seemingly never-ending milder recurrences of infection every few weeks or months.

Mary, a twenty-one-year-old secretary, came to see me because she was feeling so tired. She had been involved in a car crash when she was eighteen and was sufficiently shaken and bruised to be taken to hospital for a check-up. Nothing major was found and she was discharged the same evening. The next day she saw her GP because she had a bad headache over her eyes and felt very stiff in her back. This settled down in the next few weeks but she never felt as well as before the accident.

One year later she had a viral infection which left her exhausted; but she got over this within a month. A few months later she had a further viral attack, followed by flu-like attacks. These stopped after a couple of years. By now, however, she was so exhausted she had to give up work. A diet designed to avoid food intolerances helped but not enough to get her back to work.

She came to me with a list of symptoms, including dizziness and indigestion, a woolly feeling in her head and a very poor memory. Examination revealed extensive spasm of the spinal muscles, especially in the thoracic region. Her blood pressure was low, she had a painful hip and shoulder joints, and her stomach was very tender. Her tonsils were large and infected and there was a number of large, tender lymph nodes in her neck. Mary's tonsils were removed and I gave her my form of physiotherapy and remobilization, and treated her lymph nodes with ultrasonic waves and massage for nearly three months. By this time she felt eighty per cent on the road to recovery. After another three to four months she was back to work feeling better than she could remember. The woolly feeling in her head was the last symptom to go, and was relieved by six magnesium injections.

Some of the Main Symptoms of Chronic Fatigue Syndrome

Complete exhaustion

A large number of lymph nodes are intermingled with the sympathetic nerve centres (see figure 6.3). The latter, as we have seen in Chapter Four, control almost all the parameters of the body and are linked with the adrenalin mechanism. If a patient is suffering from low sympathetic drive, one of the main symptoms is fatigue. This is caused by the poor action of the muscle pump, leading to a build-up of oedema in the tissue spaces, which chokes the sympathetic nerve centres and lowers their efficiency. If these nerve centres become even more water-logged as a result of the inflammation of the adjacent lymph nodes, then clearly the feeling of tiredness will be even greater. In fact, it may be so great that the patient is overwhelmed by exhaustion at the slightest effort.

Wendy, thirty-eight and a keen sportswoman, came to me

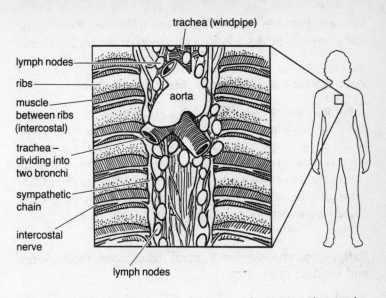

Figure 6.3 The close proximity of the sympathetic nerve chain and the lymph nodes. Clearly, if the lymph nodes are inflamed, the nerve centres will become waterlogged.

complaining of extreme fatigue. She had been a very energetic person for many years but she now felt permanently exhausted and could not understand why. As we talked, she revealed that she had suffered a bad attack of glandular fever six years previously. From then on she had never felt well. She suffered some indigestion, she slept badly, she felt very tensed up and she had times of feeling depressed. She also had fibrositic pains between her shoulder blades. On examination she had considerable spasm of the back muscles in the chest area, particularly between the shoulder blades. This is a typical picture of ME – especially as the clinical tests were normal.

After eight treatments to her back (see page 136 for a description of the treatment) she was fit and well again.

Many patients, like Wendy, suffer from a history of

fibrositis between the shoulders and mild symptoms of the low sympathetic drive before the onset of the severe illness.

Poor memory and a 'woolly' feeling in the head

Tiredness and a 'woolly' feeling are symptoms of a magnesium deficiency in the red blood cells. This may come about as a result of poor absorption due to the stomach condition, alternatively, due to stress or anxiety, the body can excrete excessive amounts. People suffering the symptoms of ME, as well as a poor memory, can be greatly helped by injections of magnesium.

Indigestion, vitamin and mineral deficiencies, food allergy and candida infestation

Another result of low sympathetic drive is indigestion. This is due to the excess acid in the stomach caused by parasympathetic over-activity. The excessive acid can inflame the stomach lining and impair the absorption of certain substances even though they may be plentiful in the diet. One of the first casualties of this is the Vitamin B group. Shortage makes the patient feel even more tired and depressed.

Whether for the same reason or not, patients suffering from Chronic Fatigue Syndrome often have a shortage of the trace elements Zinc, Magnesium and occasionally Copper and Chromium. These shortages can affect the function of the antibodies and so make it even more difficult to throw off an infection.

The inflammation of the stomach also makes it more sensitive, so certain substances which may irritate it somewhat, as we have seen in Chapter Four, can cause an allergic reaction. A patient may respond in a relatively simple way with an acute response such as a strawberry rash, or there may be a more complex reaction. This is because the effect of the allergy itself is often over-ridden for an hour or two by a massive release of the natural cortisone of the body, which is a powerful anti-allergen and gives a feeling of wellbeing. After the cortisone has worn off, the patient has a feeling of tiredness and depression.

The sad thing is that the initial feeling of wellbeing so often makes a patient suffering from Chronic Fatigue Syndrome think that the particular food to which he is allergic is his saviour and he resorts to it frequently to try and regain fitness. This is exactly what happened to me.

Ten years ago, I had become so tired for the previous year or so that I was thinking of retiring. I had a full check-up and nothing really was found to be wrong. In fact, I was told that I was very fit. Undiagnosed tiredness is a common symptom in people coming to see me so I decided to give myself a consultation. Again, nothing seemed to be the cause until I thought of food intolerance. Suddenly, I realized my problem – coffee.

I had a cup of coffee before I got out of bed in the morning; the main attraction of breakfast was coffee; my secretary virtually faced the sack if I was not greeted with a cup; at eleven I could not see another patient until I had consumed my elevenses cup; and lunch was highlighted by my post-prandial cup of coffee. This increase in consumption coincided to a large extent with the onset of my fatigue.

For this reason I became convinced that I was allergic to coffee. I stopped drinking it, but within two days I knew that I could not continue working unless I had a cup. It was not until I went on holiday that I was able to give it up after two very difficult weeks.

As explained earlier, the coffee stimulates a huge output

of cortisone, with an accompanying feeling of wellbeing. As the cortisone level drops below normal, this feeling changes to a feeling of fatigue and depression, and we feel that we must have another cup to get the feel of wellbeing back. The lack of cortisone increases until the tiredness becomes overwhelming.

In my case, after many months one cup of coffee did not result in too excessive a drop in cortisone so I was able to have an occasional cup.

If for whatever reason an allergic reaction is suspected then the patient can be put on an elimination diet which disallows all substances known to cause an allergy. Gradually foods are re-introduced one at a time so that the culprit is discovered when the patient suffers a sharp reaction. Common offenders are dairy produce, white flour and coffee. Many people choose to try this for themselves. However, for such a diet to give positive results it is important to eliminate more than one substance that might be under suspicion. Either work out all the substances that might be suspected of causing the allergy and avoid eating them or indulge in a total elimination diet that excludes all known allergens. You will probably feel particularly bad for a few days. The improvement comes after about five days when the body has cleared itself of all the offending substances. Other methods of testing for allergies including skin and blood tests can give very good results.

There may be other symptoms of an allergy such as: aches between the shoulders; pain and swelling in some joints, perhaps the fingers or a knee; swollen ankles; abdominal symptoms such as vague indigestion, bowel upsets and distention; headaches; catarrh; depression and even mental disorder.

In the same group as food allergies is candida infestation, especially of the bowel. Candida is a yeast-like fungus that is found virtually everywhere. It is normally harmless to humans but thrives in people under certain conditions, including those who are either rundown, suffering from a food allergy or Vitamin B deficiency, eating a poor diet, often containing excessive sugar and, most important, taking antibiotics to fight infection. The colonies of 'helpful' bacteria in the body that compete with candida for space and food in the body are greatly diminished by the antibiotics so the candida can take over.

The candida may well be all over the body but the place that affects the patient most is the bowel. This is yet another contributing factor in making the patient tire more easily and become very depressed. Candida produces a similar allergy to food, but unlike a food allergy the candida would be present all the time, so the cortisone becomes exhausted and permanent tiredness sets in. The irritation of the infection causes disruption of normal intestinal function, causing abdominal symptoms such as indigestion, distension and diarrhoea. Some doctors do not think that the bowel becomes involved. They think that it is the 'Candida Diet' that makes the patient feel better by unintentionally eliminating a food intolerance. This is a strict diet which forbids bread and other substances containing yeast or fungus, and sugar especially (even in the minutest quantities).

Weakness of the joints

A number of patients suffering from Chronic Fatigue Syndrome complain of weakness in a leg or arm, and even that the limb suddenly gives way at times, causing them to stumble or drop things. Again, this could be due to the malfunction of the sympathetic nervous system. It is suggested on page 149 that low sympathetic drive could cause joints to become arthritic because the normal repair after wear doesn't occur completely.

In many of the patients complaining of weak limbs there is an associated joint that is arthritic. When a joint is not in perfect working order, nature makes an attempt to give it a rest and increase its chance of healing by immobilizing it. Pain is the most obvious device, but it is also common for the nerve supply to the muscles working the joint to limit the power available. This gives the impression that the leg is heavy and not working very well, or that the arm or grip is weak. This weakness is not a neurological disorder but one of the normal mechanisms of repair.

An annoying extension of this is that, in moments of extra effort or stress, the nerves may cut off the muscle power almost completely for a brief second. This could cause the person to stumble or even fall, or to drop something they were holding in their hand. However, with correct diagnosis and treatment this can also be helped.

When Margaret, sixty-three, came to see me she said she had been suffering from arthritis for the past fifteen years. Five years ago it had become very bad and she had had her toes operated on. She said she often woke with pain in her left shoulder and also had trouble in her left hip. The main problem, however, was her left hand. It is weak and painful all the time, especially in cold weather. The first finger and wrist were the worst. She said she had recently dropped a plate of hot food when her wrist had 'given way'. Margaret had been seeing an osteopath for twenty-five years, for neck and back treatment. Margaret had migraine attacks but no indigestion.

On examination I found that her neck movements were below normal. The normal movement of the neck is most easily assessed by turning the head from side to side – the chin should just about go over the shoulder and turn in an angle of ninety degrees. If the head will only turn half this way to forty-five degrees, the movement is said to be fifty per cent of normal. Margaret's head movements were seventy per cent normal.

There was an increase of the lumbar curve and the muscles were in considerable spasm. The sixth cervical and fourth lumbar vertebrae were tender. Various joints were swollen and tender, especially the left fingers and wrist. Tests for rheumatism were negative.

My diagnosis was that she had injured her back in the past, and that the oedema from the poor muscle pump had involved the sympathetic nerve centres. As a result of this, she had faulty repair of the various joints, causing the weakness and 'giving way' of the wrist. This cleared up after fourteen more visits, when her back was treated. She also had local treatment to the various affected joints with ultrasonic waves and re-mobilization, and an anti-inflammatory drug to speed up the effect of the treatment. Although she still has slight pains at times, she sleeps well and feels stronger and better than she can ever remember.

Depression

Unfortunately depression is a common symptom of a low sympathetic drive, a viral infection, and Vitamin B and magnesium deficiencies, and it can also be endogenous (built-in) to some people. Many of the effects of Chronic Fatigue Syndrome, such as depression, may need treating separately, as they may not respond to my treatment alone. If a faulty fence at the top of a cliff results in an unfortunate person falling to the bottom, it may well not be sufficient to repair the fence. The poor victim may well require a bandage on a wound and a splint on a fracture.

Depression in the medical sense is more a feeling of being unable to get going or start doing anything. With all the causes present in the Chronic Fatigue Syndrome, depression can be the most difficult of the individual symptoms to correct. Fortunately, a majority of patients respond very well to the treatment I offer to the back and lymph nodes. However, there are a few severe and complicated cases where I believe that a comprehensive unit able to deal with all these problems is needed.

A Positive Approach

What you can do to help yourself

1. Try to keep as fit as possible – it is very important to keep going. Take the maximum exercise possible without causing excessive fatigue – little and often is the motto.

2. Try modifying your diet. Often coffee, dairy produce (and this means *all* produce – cheese, yoghurt, etc.) and/or white flour can upset people. Sugar is often a cause of trouble and, if so, needs to be eliminated as completely as possible. Remember, it takes about five days to get the last traces of sugar and other foods out of the body, so just one lapse on the fourth day and you have to begin again. Think of the time gone as an investment not to be frittered away.

If an elimination diet is needed for a complete assessment of food sensitivities, it would probably be better to purchase a book on the subject for complete details (see page 242 for my suggestions).

3. Replace trace elements. These can be taken separately as Vitamin B tablets or fluid (I think that the synthetic ones are superior). Vitamin B12 tablets are better taken separately. Vitamins A, D and C are also often a help in increasing resistance to infection. Try Vitamins A and D as cod or halibut liver oil in the recommended dosage, and Vitamin C up to 2 grams daily (or one twice a day to avoid diarrhoea). Among other elements

often needed are Iron, Magnesium, Manganese, Chromium and Zinc. These can be taken separately (Zinc should always be taken on its own at night), or in a combined form with Vitamin C. There is a pill that has been created especially for ME sufferers; it is available from Lambert's (see page 244). Other remedies such as Royal Jelly may help, but are of questionable value.

General diet control may also be of assistance. Eat each group of foods separately – one meal carbohydrates – another protein. Some people find that avoiding meat helps them. Often only red meat needs to be abandoned.

4. Massage to the neck and back by a friend or relative can often help. It should be firm and given for ten to twenty minutes. Massage to the lymph nodes in the neck will often help get over the infectious part of the illness.

5. Contact one of the helpful associations for support and advice about what your own doctor can do (see page 244 for details of some organizations). Then,

- Suggest physical medicine to the neck and thoracic spine as detailed in the last chapter of this book, 'A Note For Your Therapist', (page 216).
- Discuss with your doctor the possibility of receiving intravenous Vitamin B two to three times a week.
- Have trace elements assessed (red cell Magnesium included) and replace any found in short supply. *Note*: The acceptable lower margin of normal is not adequate in people suffering from ME, especially in the case of Iron. This should be raised to the top level of normality. If short, red cell Magnesium needs to be replenished by weekly intra-muscular injections.
- The depression often needs treating as it can become severe and obstruct the whole recovery. Anti-depress-

ant drugs may be needed for a few weeks but can usually be given up shortly after the patient begins to feel altogether better.

- A number of patients who only feel moderately improved by all these measures will require Nystatin by mouth. It needs to be in a pure form and *not* taken as a tablet. The powder is probably best, but capsules are available (rather expensive). The dose needs to be started fairly low, gradually increasing as advised by your doctor. This needs to be continued for at least two to three months.

- General and moral support are a great help to the sufferer. It is demoralizing to feel ill and to have your life in tatters − and then to be told that there is nothing wrong.

Hopefully, this description of ME or the Chronic Fatigue Syndrome will be of some help to sufferers. Certainly, it is my experience that the majority of patients can be helped to return to a full and rewarding life. Indeed, many admit they haven't felt so fit and healthy for many years.

The next chapter looks at each symptom associated with sympathetic malfunction separately, as individual diseases.

7

TAKING YOUR BACK SERIOUSLY

*Your back – an unsuspected
cause of illness*

When beginning the siege of Madrid in the Spanish Civil War, General Mola said, 'I have four columns operating against Madrid and a fifth column inside.' In this chapter, we ask the question – is the spinal column a 'fifth column'?

We have dealt with back pain and the problems which a patient clearly associates with their back. In this chapter we will look at some diseases that are, in my view, often caused by back problems but are seldom recognized as such. As a result, patients are all too often given symptomatic treatment that does nothing to help the underlying trouble. If treatment is directed at the basic cause then a more effective and lasting relief can be obtained.

The individual diseases we will discuss in this chapter are determined by which ganglion, or group of nerve centres, is affected by the oedema. Oedema, as you will remember from page 37, can be caused by muscle spasm due to a spinal injury. In Chapter Five, we discussed the Hyposympathetic Tone Syndrome (HST), in which a number of nerve centres are involved, giving rise to several symptoms. In themselves these symptoms are often not very severe. However, when only a single ganglion is affected, the symptoms are usually much more pronounced. For example, someone suffering from low sympathetic drive may have vague indigestion as one of his symptoms. When only one ganglion is involved, there is usually only one dominant condition and it is correspondingly more pronounced, for example, a gastric or duodenal ulcer.

It is probably easier to consider the diseases brought about by back trouble by looking at what happens when the various ganglia are not functioning efficiently. To do this, I will start at the top of the nerve chain and work downwards. For each ganglion I shall describe its relevant function and then show how and why problems can occur. Before continuing, however, it is important that you fully understand my theory on the cause of back pain and related diseases. If you wish to refresh your memory you should re-read Chapter Three.

Stellate Ganglion

This group of ganglia, or little brains, lies at the base of the neck. The two main functions are:

- to control the amount of blood that passes through the arteries to the head and arms; and
- to monitor the repair of tissues. In the context of this book, this applies particularly to the joints and tendons in the arm.

Now let's look at these functions in more detail to discover what happens when something goes wrong with the stellate ganglion.

MIGRAINE HEADACHES

The first function to be discussed is that of controlling the flow of blood through the arteries to the head and arms. Arteries are vessels which carry blood out from the heart to the tissues of the body. A relatively small amount of blood must supply the whole body. In order for this to happen, the body contains an almost unbelievably complicated mechanism similar to irrigation.

The arteries have circular muscles in their walls which can vary the internal diameter. Contracting these muscles lessens this diameter, or in smaller vessels, closes the hole off completely. The use of this property enables the body to make a relatively small amount of circulating blood (i.e., about eight pints) supply a large area by an incredibly sophisticated form of irrigation. It has been estimated that with modern technology if we were to try and construct a human being we would need at least seventy pints of blood to perform the same function.

Sensors detect when an area is short of supplies and full of waste products and accordingly send impulses to the appropriate autonomic centres. These then open up the vessels supplying the affected area until the situation is corrected. The centre then closes the supply to that area and opens it up in another needy place. When the system is working efficiently, there is complete control of the amount of blood that goes to any one part of the body. Local controlling mechanisms also have an influence on this mechanism.

If the ganglion malfunctions then it may cause the arterial walls to contract too hard, and to narrow abnormally the internal diameter and even to shut off smaller ones completely over a wide area.

The cause of migraine

If someone has suffered a previous injury involving the base of the neck – perhaps in a car accident or on the sports field – then the stellate ganglion may be affected by the ensuing local oedema. Eventually this group of nerve centres will reach a critical point as a result of poor drainage brought about by muscle spasm. Under these conditions, it may malfunction and close off the circulation to the brain, so depriving it of oxygen and essential nutrients. The brain, however, cannot survive very long without oxygen so this arterial spasm is violently over-ridden, causing the artery to dilate over a large area of its distribution. The brain becomes flooded and as it is held within a rigid structure – the skull – this causes a considerable rise in pressure. The result of this is a condition called 'migraine headache'.

The lack of blood to the brain during the arterial spasm upsets the function of various nerve centres in the brain. This causes a number of corresponding symptoms, such as visual disturbance, a pins-and-needles sensation in, say, an arm or hand, and other symptoms a patient learns to associate with the onset of a headache. The next stage is the flooding of the brain which, due to the rise of pressure in the skull, causes headache, sickness, usually severe vomiting, and various other symptoms such as sensitivity to light and sound.

The arterial spasm is widely recognized as the cause of a migraine and the mainstay of treatment is to give drugs (containing ergotamine, which constrict the arteries to limit the flooding of the brain) at the moment of onset. Analgesics such as aspirin, paracetamol or co-proxamal may help to relieve the pain, and anti-sickness drugs such as metoclopramide can be combined with the others to help control nausea and vomiting. A new injection of a serotonin inhibitor, Imigran, is very effective at stopping a headache at any stage of the attack. Drugs given to prevent attacks have to be given over a period of time; these are betablockers, such as propalalol, and seratonin antagonists, such as pitzotifen or rivotril. None of these drugs cures the disease – they are merely different ways

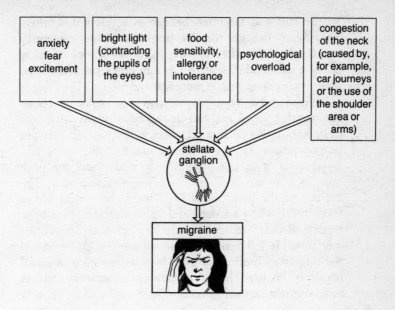

Figure 7.1 Some of the stimuli which trigger a migraine.

of minimizing the effect of the headaches. Figure 7.1 shows the triggers of migraine on the stellate ganglion.

As I have just discussed, I believe that the stellate ganglion is involved and that by treating the underlying problem in the back, rather than the symptoms, it is possible to give permanent relief. The success of my theory is shown by Richard and Christine, whose stories are told below.

Richard, a fifty-six-year-old architect, told me he had began suffering from migraine headaches at around five years of age. At first they were infrequent but they became more and more intense and frequent. By the time he was ten he was having them every few days and he had even begun to make himself sick as he found that this aborted the headache. Things had improved somewhat over the years

143

but he still had migraine headaches severely and often. They were brought on by bright sunshine, becoming excessively tired, after playing games at school or fairly heavy exercise and, later on in life, after gardening and moderate or long motor journeys.

Richard tired very easily, and had some fibrositis between his shoulders and at the base of his neck. On examination, his neck movements were about seventy per cent of normal. There was intense spasm of the paravertebral muscles from the occiput, which is where the neck muscles join the skull, to the lower thoracic area. The muscles at the base of the skull were very tender. After seven visits, when his neck and upper thoracic spine were treated, Richard still had slight headaches but no actual migraine. He left feeling on top of the world. However, the migraines returned a year later following a stressful period of his life. He had three more treatments and has had no further trouble since.

Like many migraine sufferers, Christine, a thirty-four-year-old mother of three, has to be in a dark room when she has an attack as she feels sick and is upset by the slightest sound or light.

Christine came to me because she had been suffering from severe headaches for nearly twenty years. They were relieved by ergotamine tablets. On two occasions a cluster of these headaches had become so severe she was put into hospital. She had been given many drugs and diets but none of these had really helped. She tired very easily, had postural dizzy spells, indigestion, low blood pressure and generally felt washed out.

When I examined Christine, I found an extreme tenderness just under the skull. The muscles were so tight or hard in spasm that the extra pressure from my fingers was enough to produce the pain. Her neck movements were seventy per cent of normal. She had seven visits, during which time her neck and thoracic spine were treated to relieve the neck problem, which then improved the muscle pump. As the oedema began to reduce, the headaches began to subside. After three to four months, they gave her no further trouble.

If you are a migraine sufferer you will sympathize with Richard and Christine. You too may have been searching for many years for some clues as to why you suffer attacks and what you can do to prevent them.

If the stellate ganglion is indeed the usual cause of a migraine headache then the theory will provide answers to many of your questions and explain why certain factors are likely to precipitate a crisis. The most common times you get a migraine are when you wake up in the morning; after eating certain foods such as chocolate; in bright light, especially in spring sunshine; when you are tired, anxious or excited; after car journeys; and after exercise of the shoulder girdle such as typing or tennis.

Why is it that as soon as I get excited I have a migraine attack?

Anything that would stimulate the stellate ganglion itself or the whole sympathetic system is a possible trigger. We have already seen that fear, tension and anxiety stimulate the sympathetic adrenalin system to prepare the person to cope efficiently in an emergency. Thus, these emotions are often found to be the cause of a migraine. Excitement can also be added to the list.

Under primitive conditions, excitement did not exist in the way we know it today. That's to say, there was no such thing as excitement at the prospect of some happy happening, such as going out on a special date. It is only since humans have developed the power of speech and communication that we can look forward to events. This being so, excitement is muddled with fear by the subconscious and both produce adrenalin. As far as the stellate ganglion are concerned, a person reacts in the same way whether they are excited at the thought of a forthcoming party or terrified as they face a mugger with a sharp knife.

Excitement is a common cause of migraine. Many sufferers get an attack just before they are about to go on holiday or when they are about to do something they have been looking forward to for some while.

Why do I so often get a migraine on a sunny day?

The pupil of the eye is to some extent controlled by the stellate ganglion, which allows it to contract with the stimulation of bright light. So when the weather suddenly becomes sunny with bright clear skies – especially at the beginning of spring – this can trigger off attacks. It is not clear why the April sun causes migraine reactions; it is possible that after winter, the bright sunshine may be more difficult to adjust to, than later, when the brain becomes more used to the light.

Do some foods cause migraine headaches?

Certain foods do indeed trigger attacks. Many people find that chocolate provokes a migraine. When you eat food which is difficult to digest or to which you are allergic, the stomach needs an extra supply of blood to help it cope. Blood is diverted to the stomach from other areas. If the stellate ganglion is malfunctioning, instead of a mild contraction diminishing the blood supply to the brain, a spasm takes place, cutting it off altogether – and that precipitates a headache.

Unfortunately, the same condition that makes a person prone to migraines also makes him or her particularly susceptible to food sensitivities. This is because the nerve centre that controls acid to the stomach is near the stellate ganglion and so is often involved to some extent in the water-logging. As a result, there may be an excess of acid in the stomach, which can make it at least slightly inflamed. This produces conditions whereby sensitivities and later allergies to food can readily come about.

Such food sensitivities can be a common cause of triggering a headache, but they are only one of the possible causes. Fortunately, if the excess acid disappears, as the conditions causing the migraine are treated, the sensitivity to the food will often settle down and thus not cause any more headaches. It is, however, sometimes necessary to take active steps to deal with the food allergy.

My migraines often start after a long car journey. Why is this?

Increased local oedema can upset the stellate ganglion enough to trigger off an attack. During a car journey, for example, your neck has a lot of work keeping your very heavy head upright against the inertia of braking, accelerating and cornering. To cope with the extra effort, your neck muscles need a considerably increased supply of blood. Unfortunately, during a car journey there is very little actual movement of the head and so the muscle pump is relatively ineffective. This results in a build-up of oedema in the base of neck, thus upsetting the stellate ganglion and causing the onset of a headache.

For some reason I often get a migraine several hours after chopping up wood. Can you explain why?

Extra activity with the arms – such as chopping up wood, playing some games or lifting weights – increases the muscular activity in the shoulders and neck and likewise increases the arterial supply. During the actual work, the muscle pump is quite effective and the tissue fluids remain at a reasonable pressure. Unfortunately, the greatly increased supply of blood to the muscles does not immediately die back once the work is completed but fades away over a period of time. Whilst the blood supply is still excessive it floods the neck area after you have stopped the activity and this may trigger a migraine even some hours later.

I've been told that migraine is a psychological disease. Is this true?

A number of people believe migraine is a psychological disorder. It is my belief that migraine is a purely physical disease brought about by the causes just discussed. It is common, however, to have a psychological overlay superimposed on a physical condition. This is a rather long-winded way of saying that conditioned reflexes develop. To explain this, I shall use the example of a dog at feeding time. If you ring a bell and then feed a dog he will associate the food with the bell and come whenever you ring the bell. Now if, after a long period of time, you stop feeding the dog but continue to ring the bell the dog will react as follows. First he will come whenever you ring it, but after a while he will become more reluctant and then not come at all.

In humans, the subconscious can note that a headache prevents you from doing something you find unpleasant, such as visiting an unpopular aunt or from going to school when you have not completed your homework. So when a similar occasion arises your subconscious may mimic a headache – which you believe to be a genuine migraine – as an escape mechanism. In some people, the induced headaches can actually outnumber the genuine attacks. Fortunately, if the physical cause can be disposed of (as when you stop feeding the dog) then the psychological attacks gradually fade out and cease to be a problem.

ARTHRITIS OF THE SHOULDER AND HAND

The second function of the stellate ganglion is that it monitors control of the repair of tissues. In the context of this book, this particularly applies to the joints and tendons in the arm. This repair mechanism is normally very efficient.

People who complain of painful joints are often told that it is because they are wearing out. 'What do you expect at your age!' I see a number of people under the age of twenty with joint pains, very many in middle age and probably a similar number of older people. At what point in their life would a person be insulted if they were told they are wearing out? Based on my experience I do not believe that under normal circumstances we actually wear out during our lifetime.

If you bought a very fine car and ran it twelve or more hours a day, every day of the year, I put it to you that the bearings would probably be very worn after, say, five years. One would assume that the joints in the body are only moderately superior vis-à-vis a car so that they would be expected to show marked wear after ten or fifteen years. The fact that there is no wear is because each time a joint is used and becomes worn, sensors in it send impulses to the appropriate sympathetic ganglion, which initiates the multiplication of cells in it, helped by local reactions, until all wear has been corrected. As your repair slows down through age, so does your level of activity to match it. I believe that if a joint becomes actually worn, it is because something, somewhere, has gone wrong with the repair mechanism.

Emily first felt discomfort in her left knee twelve years before coming to see me, when she was sixty-six years old. The discomfort only occurred randomly, and as it had not stopped her getting around she didn't seek medical advice. But around her seventy-third birthday the pain started in her other knee as well and this became much worse, beginning to make walking difficult. A consultant told her that it was arthritis because of her age and an operation might be needed if it became very bad. Physiotherapy helped a little, but the pain in the knee slowly became more obtrusive.

She told me she had suffered from mild lumbago at times for over twenty years. On examination I found her two knees were swollen and painful with limited movement. Her back had almost no lumbar curve and there was a considerable amount of spasm of the muscles caused by an old injury that had bruised the facet joints.

After eleven visits, during which time her lumbar spine was treated to improve the damaged facet joints, the spasm was gradually resolved. As this happened, she began to feel much better and her knees began to improve as the function of the lumbar sympathetic ganglion was restored. She had three visits over the next three months, by which time the knees were no longer swollen. However, she still feels some discomfort in her right knee when going up stairs. Unfortunately, I can suggest no reason for this.

As the success of the treatment for Emily's knees shows, a joint will only start to wear if something goes wrong with the repair mechanism. Once this can be made to work effectively again then the joint will be restored to good order, whatever the age of the person. There does, however, come a time when a patient cannot recover with this treatment. A normal joint has very smooth surfaces of cartilage and a special fluid which oils the joint and reduces the friction (and therefore wear) to a very low level.

As the cartilage wears and becomes slightly rough it acts as a mild sandpaper to the other side of the joint and so the wear in it increases considerably. As the joint becomes more worn the increased wear with each movement goes up dramatically until a stage is reached where the ability to replace cells is exceeded by the destruction of them. It is now no longer possible for the joint to recover but fortunately this occurs only after a great deal of wear has taken place.

The repair of the tissues in the shoulder and arms is influenced by the stellate ganglion. If it is not functioning properly, the repair of the joint is somewhat inadequate. There may be no initial symptoms but over a period of time the wear becomes significant. There comes a point when either the wear has got to a critical level or the person does something unusual or undertakes an activity that involves the joint in extra exertion. In either case, the stellate ganglion is made aware that it is a year or so behind with its repair mechanism and is prompted into action.

Emergency action

Instead of speeding up repair in a gentle symptomless way as it would normally do, the stellate ganglion panics and rings the alarm bells. The emergency repair mechanism is immediately put to work. This results in what we call an inflammatory reaction, where the blood supply is greatly increased to the affected tissues in the shoulder and hands. The extra oxygen and nutrients from this new supply of blood makes the joints considerably better for a short time but the relief is only temporary. The emergency reaction also creates a sensation of pain, making the patient more aware of the joints in order to prevent him from using them. This increased awareness of the shoulder or hand creates painful sensations under conditions that would not have caused any trouble before the first attack.

To illustrate this point, let me compare the stellate ganglion to a farm manager in charge of the day-to-day running of a large farm. If you are a prosperous farm owner you may well employ a manager to look after the ordinary running, repair and maintenance of the farm without necessarily referring back to you. The stellate ganglion is the manager of the upper part of the body and it will perform these functions without there being any conscious awareness of the things needing to be done or even the fact that they are being repaired.

If, however, a neighbour telephones you to complain that his prize dahlias have been trampled to the dust by your cows, the chances are you would make an irate phone call to your manager to ask what is going on. He will explain that a short length of fence had fallen down allowing the cows to escape. You may well be extremely annoyed by this inefficiency and insist on being informed if so much as a stick comes out of any fence in future.

So, after this incident the manager will inform you of trivial matters that would previously have been dealt with without consultation. In the same way, once the body has been made aware of the shoulder and hand, it reacts to even the most minor change in conditions. Just as the manager telephones the owner of the farm so the conscious brain is made aware of each episode by messages producing the sensation of pain.

Alexander, a forty-seven-year-old teacher, came to me complaining of rheumatoid arthritis. His fingers and wrists were swollen and painful and other joints, particularly his shoulders, had become fleetingly troublesome but had improved on their own. Arthritic blood tests were all negative.

On examination, there was considerable spasm of the paravertebral muscles throughout his back. When I asked about any previous injuries, he remembered that he'd had a bad fall from a horse twenty-one years before and had been suffering from slight backache fairly frequently for about six years. He had been to an osteopath on a number of occasions, both for backache and for pain in his left shoulder. He said he had been feeling tired and unwell for around six years.

I diagnosed that the fall off the horse had damaged his paravertebral joints and that he had had a steady build-up of oedema in his back tissues that had become bad enough for him to have a drop in his sympathetic drive, six years before. This caused the fatigue which started at that time. Even in those periods when extra activity had reduced the oedema enough to eliminate the pain, the problem in the back remained the same, and the brain continued to be conscious of the tiredness. As well as the tiredness, the low sympathetic drive also caused the problem in the fingers, which remained continuously painful.

When he first felt pain, he remembers his fingers being quite swollen around the joints. Alexander had seven visits and the treatment with physical medicine I gave to his back relieved the spasm to a great extent. The fingers were about seventy per cent better and he said he was feeling much improved in himself. Three months later his fingers had almost recovered but felt painful, especially the day after he had used them a lot. Six months later all the pain had gone and Alexander said he just couldn't believe how well he felt.

If the stellate ganglion is not working efficiently the fingers can be very painful. This is because they are in constant use. If the normal repair mechanism is not functioning properly then the build-up of wear over the years will reach a critical point and the alarm bells will start ringing. The emergency repair mechanism is set in motion, which causes an abnormal reaction of swelling and pain. As time passes, the fingers can become increasingly painful, especially if the person uses the hand a great deal.

Charlotte, sixty-one, was at her wits' end when she came to see me. Three years before she had been mugged and when her attackers snatched her handbag she clung on so tightly that the first finger of her right hand was dislocated. She said she had suffered pain in the finger right up to the elbow ever since and this could be very bad at times. Her hand was very weak and did not seem to respond to any treatment.

As we talked, she revealed that she had been involved in a car crash fifteen years before and had suffered a fairly severe whiplash injury. Her neck had been stiff on and off since. She was also suffering from high blood pressure.

She could not straighten the first finger of her right hand. The knuckles were very tender and her hand was so weak she could not make a fist. Her neck movements were restricted and there was considerable swelling at the base. Tension resulting from this unpleasant episode may well have further tightened the neck and shoulder muscles in the 'fight' reaction (see pages 104–6), and further aggravated the condition.

On palpation, I found there was spasm of the paravertebral muscles from the skull to the mid-thoracic region and the sixth cervical vertebra was very tender.

I concluded that although the long-standing neck trouble had been reasonably stable for some time; it had flared up after the mugging, which had also damaged the joints in her hand. I decided that the hand was not repairing itself owing to defective monitoring of repair as the oedema around the stellate ganglion had interfered with its function. It responded well to treatment of the neck area, and when I saw her a year later for another problem, she said the hand had remained symptom-free.

As this case shows, treatment of the neck area will usually produce a marked and fairly rapid improvement in shoulder and hand problems, even to the point of complete relief, in most people. Curiously, shoulder problems usually occur in people in their twenties to forties and the fingers start to give trouble thereafter.

FROZEN SHOULDER

A frozen shoulder is a special version of inflammation associated with the malfunctioning of the stellate ganglion. This is a very painful state of the shoulder which causes throbbing and in some cases reduces movement almost to nothing. Once the original crisis in the nerve centre is over, the trouble usually repairs itself over a period of some months and the shoulder gets better. However, active treatment to correct the stellate ganglion can speed up the recovery time to weeks rather than months or a year.

TENNIS ELBOW

Another problem caused by an inefficient maintenance system is tennis elbow. The affected muscle is attached at one end to the arm bone (the humerus) just above the elbow on the thumb side. It runs down the forearm and then attaches at the other end just above the wrist. If there is even a slight weakness in the maintenance system, this muscle is vulnerable to damage.

The condition got its name because a backhand tennis shot puts considerable strain on the muscle at the place where it is fixed to the bone, just above the elbow, and often causes the problem. Muscles may be attached to a bone over a wide area, or form a single hard wire called a tendon, and this is attached to the bone. Tendons form where a bulk of muscle would interfere with the freedom of movement of a joint, or where the muscle is more conveniently situated a distance away from the second place to which it is attached, such as the muscles in the forearm which go into a long tendon that actually moves the fingers (which are a long way from the muscle and which are too small to have such big muscles across the actual finger joints themselves). This muscle attaches over a wide area and some of the fibres may become detached. This causes acute pain at the elbow whenever the wrist is turned, as the twisting action is brought about by contracting the damaged muscle. Although called tennis elbow, many other activities can, of course, bring about the same injury. It is a persistent condition and tends to recur even if, as with John, whose case I am about to relate, it is put right with injections of cortisone or other treatments. The simplest way to offer permanent relief is to treat the errant stellate ganglion.

John, fifty-three, an enthusiastic sportsman, had started to have bad tennis elbow about six years before he came for a consultation. At the time, he had been given a cortisone injection with immediate, complete relief. Three years later, the pain started again and he had further injections. This time there was some relief and he was able to resume playing tennis. However, in the past eighteen months the trouble had become very severe and he got no relief from cortisone.

He told me that his neck had been mildly troublesome following a skiing accident twelve years before but it had never required any treatment. He also had very mild indigestion at times.

On examination, I could feel a small knot just above the right elbow which was accompanied by the typical very tender area. His neck movements were almost normal but there was considerable spasm of the muscles from below the skull to the middle of the thoracic area. It was this that was causing oedema in the region of the stellate ganglion, causing his indigestion and delaying the healing of the tear in the muscle at the elbow.

John had seven sessions of treatment to his neck, and as this improved, so slowly did the elbow. A year later, it became uncomfortable again and three more visits were needed. Repeated treatment was needed after a trouble-free two years but since then the problem has not recurred.

A very similar condition at the other side of the elbow is known as golfer's elbow. In this instance, another muscle is torn at the point where it fixes to the bone just above the elbow, but on the other side. This is also caused by problems at the base of the neck and can be treated in the same way as tennis elbow. I have not seen a single case of tennis or golfer's elbow without accompanying neck (and therefore back) trouble.

Clifford had had bad tennis elbow twelve years before his first visit to me. An injection of cortisone had completely stopped the pain, until four years later when he made a bad backhand at tennis and the trouble recurred. He had another two injections of cortisone, which made it feel better but not completely right. Later still, he had physiotherapy with little improvement. An osteopath made it feel better but it kept on relapsing.

When I saw him he volunteered that he had had neck trouble since being in a motor car that was hit in the back, jerking his neck. The accident had taken place eight years before his first pain in the elbow.

He had eleven treatments to his neck, when the elbow was about seventy-five per cent better. In the following twelve weeks it disappeared completely.

Two years later he had a twinge of pain and returned. His neck muscle spasm had returned slightly. He had three more visits to get rid of this, and has had no further pain since.

CARPAL TUNNEL SYNDROME

Another tissue-maintenance problem is a disease called Carpal Tunnel Syndrome, with symptoms including pain, numbness or pins and needles and weakness in the thumb, first finger and the near side of the middle finger. Although mostly below the wrist, the pain can radiate up the arm towards the elbow. It is caused by a thickening of the ligament that strengthens the wrist on its palm side. This ligament is a thick band that runs from one side of the wrist to the other. Passing through a tunnel in the ligament is the median nerve that supplies the hand and fingers both with sensation and muscle control.

If the stellate ganglion is not working at its best, then this large ligament may not be properly maintained. In an attempt to give itself the extra strength needed due to this situation the ligament begins to thicken. This can result in the median nerve to the thumb, first and half the middle finger becoming pinched as it goes through its tunnel known as the carpal tunnel. It is the pinched nerve that gives rise to the symptoms known as Carpal Tunnel Syndrome (see figure 7.2).

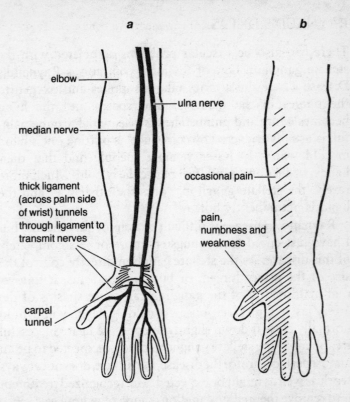

Figure 7.2 Carpal Tunnel Syndrome. Diagram *a* shows the thickening ligament, on the thumb side, pinching the nerve, causing pain and numbness. Diagram *b* shows the distribution of pain and numbness.

If the condition is not too bad, it can be treated by improving the circulation around the stellate ganglion. If, however, it is very severe or long established, then it may be necessary to operate and slit the ligament along the line of the carpal tunnel and thus free the nerve from the pinching effect. This is a very simple, effective cure.

RAYNAUD'S DISEASE

There can also be vascular problems associated with the stellate ganglion. One of the most common is Raynaud's Disease where the arteries taking supplies and oxygen to the tissues in the hand go into spasm and the hand becomes white and numb. The disease, which can be painful, is usually triggered by cold, such as putting one's hand in cold water. In lesser versions, people find that their hands, or just one hand, feel particularly cold. Much more rarely, the stellate ganglion works the other way and the hand is permanently hot.

Raynaud's Disease is difficult to help by any means, but I have just cured two youngsters more or less completely of this disease. As the stellate ganglion directly control the size of the artery lumen, or bore, in the arms, it follows that malfunction of the ganglion can cause spasms of the artery as a faulty response to cold – when you would normally close it down slightly to conserve heat. Successful treatment to the stellate ganglion could be expected to be an almost perfect cure for the disease, but, in fact, does not always work as well as might be expected. The recognized treatment is to remove the stellate ganglion completely; however, since the sympathetic chain tends to reform, the disease returns.

Splanchnic Ganglion

The next group of nerve centres to be considered is the splanchnic ganglion, which lies in the middle of the thoracic spine (see figure 7.3, page 163). The two main functions are:

- to control the amount of acid and movements of the stomach; and

● to control the blood supply to the stomach.

INDIGESTION AND FLATULENCE

Indigestion is the inability to put a square meal into a round stomach.

The first function of the splanchnic ganglion to be considered is the control of the amount of acid and movements of the stomach. To be strictly accurate, it opposes the vagus nerve, which as we discussed in Chapter Five, is part of the parasympathetic nervous system. The vagus controls the digestive system.

When food is swallowed it passes down the eating tube (or oesophagus) into the stomach. At the entrance to the stomach is a ring of powerful muscles that relax to allow the food to enter and then contract to prevent the food and acid returning into the oesophagus. The food stays in the stomach as long as is necessary for the digestive processes in it to be completed. It is therefore necessary for food to be prevented from entering the first part of the small intestine – the duodenum – until the right moment. The duodenum (meaning twelve), is, as its name implies, twelve inches long. A second ring of muscles completely blocks the exit from the stomach by contracting until the next stage of digestion is about to start. The muscle or sphyncter, as it is called, then relaxes so some of the stomach contents can flow into the intestine.

The vagus nerve is in a state of balance with the sympathetic nervous system. Each puts out a 'voltage' which under neutral conditions cancels the other out and maintains a healthy harmony. If, however, a person has back trouble in the middle of the thoracic spine – and remember, he may not be aware of this – this will cause a partial failure of the muscle pump, leading to a build-up of oedema in the affected area. This may well depress the activity of the splanchnic ganglion, causing it to malfunction.

Upsetting the balance

This malfunction of the splanchnic ganglion causes an excess of acid in the stomach. Under resting conditions, if a person is not eating anything and is in a tranquil state, little acid is produced in the stomach. If, however, the parasympathetic pull is less opposed by the diminished sympathetic drive, the balance shifts in its favour and excessive acid is produced in the stomach even when there is no food present.

As I explained earlier, it helps to picture the vagus nerve and sympathetic nervous system as two teams in an equal tug-of-war contest. If one member of a team is removed, then his team would no longer be a match for the other and the mark on the rope would be pulled relentlessly across the line. In the case of the stomach, an inequality on either side results in acid and digestive juices continuing to be secreted even after food has been fully digested. Also, the stomach carries on churning and the valves both to the oesophagus and the duodenum possibly become a little on the slack side. See figure 7.3, which illustrates the close relationship between the vagus nerve and the digestive system.

- In the earlier stages of imbalance, this results in mild indigestion. The most common symptom is that the patient nibbles all day in a subconscious attempt to mop up the acid in the stomach.
- In a more advance condition the inflammation of the stomach wall caused by the extra acid will make the patient suffer a loss of appetite. This is the body's way of trying to rest the inflamed system. What seems

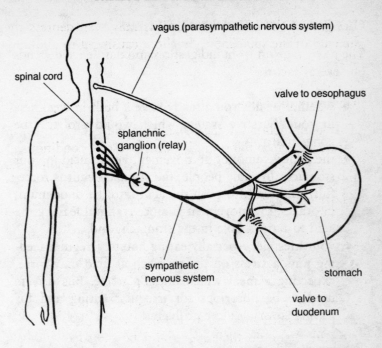

Figure 7.3 The nerve supply to the stomach. The parasympathetic nervous system initiates all digestive processes, following digestion from start to finish. The sympathetic nervous system turns off the stomach when no food is present – or when the body is experiencing fright or stress.

like flatulence is also a common symptom at this stage as the patient swallows air in a subconscious attempt to keep the inflamed membranes apart and so stop them sticking together and irritating each other.

Treatment to the back in the area of the splanchnic ganglion will almost always clear up any indigestion and flatulence by restoring its balance with the parasympathetic nervous system.

GASTRIC AND DUODENAL ULCERS

The next stage on from indigestion and flatulence depends on several factors:

- whether or not you already have a built-in weakness in your digestive system which would probably be congenital;
- the relative amount of movement versus acid in your stomach. In some people, the stomach churns forcefully and tends to push the acid into the duodenum; in others, the movement is more tranquil leaving the acid to burn a hole in the stomach; and
- your lifestyle, especially eating habits. Irregular feeding puts a stress on the stomach as acid may form, expecting a meal which doesn't arrive. Bus drivers used to be notorious for irregular eating and for having stomach-ulcer problems.

A gastric ulcer results when there are mild stomach contractions, allowing the acids to stay there longer. They will eventually burn a hole in the stomach lining, causing an ulcer.

A duodenal ulcer arises when the stomach contractions are more dominant and the acid is squeezed through a valve called the pyloric sphyncter (pylorus means gatekeeper) into the duodenum (intestine). As the duodenum normally contains alkaline juices it is not used to coping with the acid juices and a hole is burned in its lining.

Tension is often blamed as a major contributor to a gastric or duodenal ulcer. My contention is that this tensed-up state is actually part of the same problem that causes the ulcer. Let me explain my reasoning. You are by now familiar with the effects of a low sympathetic drive, as discussed in previous chapters. One of the body's reactions is to try and lift the drive through a compensatory mechanism in the brain, which stimulates the anxiety/fright centre. As a result, the patient feels anxious and tensed up. It is probable that the state of anxiety will stimulate the sympathetic/adrenalin system and will thus actually help to switch off the secretion of acid and the movements of the stomach and so may in fact help reduce the effect of the inflammation of the stomach.

Alternatively, tranquillizers are often helpful in the treatment of the ulcers because they cause a relaxation of the muscle spasm in the back and this diminishes the low sympathetic drive.

Both gastric and duodenal ulcers can usually be cured successfully by treatment to the lower neck and the upper half of the thoracic spine, which corrects the malfunction of the splanchnic ganglion. At this point it must be stressed that if the indigestion is severe or an ulcer present these should be investigated and treated in an orthodox manner at the same time. Clearly, serious complications could occur before the back treatment has effected any major improvement.

HIATUS HERNIA

Hiatus hernia is the other condition greatly aggravated by the malfunction of the splanchnic ganglion. The most prominent symptom is a burning sensation under the breast bone, which is particularly noticeable at night or any other time the patient may lie down. The symptoms of simple indigestion are often attributed to an hiatus hernia, if one is found when the stomach is X-rayed. However, indigestion itself is seldom caused by an hiatus hernia.

As figure 7.4 shows, the diaphragm divides near the backbone to allow the big arteries and veins, the oesophagus and other structures to pass from the chest into the

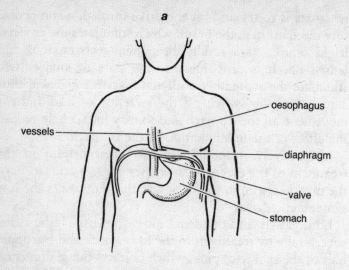

Figure 7.4 Diagram *a* shows a normal oesophagus, passing through the close-fitting hole in the diaphragm. Diagram *b* shows a hiatus hernia, where the valve has become stretched, and food and acid regurgitate into the oesophagus – inflaming it and causing a burning pain under the lower part of the breast bone.

abdomen and vice versa. If the diaphragm has a larger hole than is necessary for this purpose, some of the stomach may well pass through the gap into the chest cavity, dividing itself into two parts shaped rather like an hourglass. This is an hiatus hernia. Obviously, the normal function of the stomach is interfered with. In particular, it causes acid to pass up into the eating tube when the patient is lying down, hence the discomfort at night.

Treatment to the area of the splanchnic ganglion will tighten the muscular ring, or valve, to the oesophagus and may go a long way to relieving the symptoms of regurgitation caused by the hiatus hernia. It will, of course, also lessen the resting acid levels and thus help to relieve any indigestion that may be present.

166

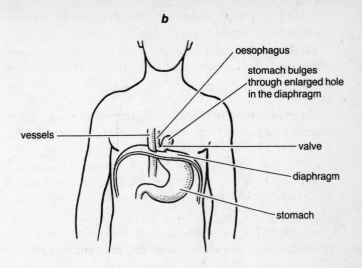

ABDOMINAL MIGRAINE

The second function of the splanchnic ganglion is to control the supply of blood to the abdomen. If the nerve centres are not functioning as they should be then this may cause the artery to the intestines to go into cramp, causing a severe abdominal pain, usually accompanied by nausea and a feeling of general ill-health. This is an abdominal migraine. It almost always responds well to treatment to the mid-thoracic area with physical medicine.

Mary, thirty-four, complained of abdominal migraine. The first attack had been just over three years previously, and had begun about an hour after lunch. She had suffered severe cramp-like pain in a wide area of the abdomen and she had felt unwell and nauseous.

The next attack was around two years later and was similar. She then suffered two more attacks during the next year. They all began around half an hour to two hours after eating and there was no obvious reason for them. She had been fully investigated for an abdominal problem in hospital but everything appeared to be normal.

Mary said she had been feeling rather low and had been tiring easily for several years. She had mild indigestion at times and a very occasional, slight ache between the shoulders.

On examination of the stomach, I found nothing abnormal. The back, however, showed considerable spasm of the paravertebral muscles in the mid-chest region. Her blood pressure was on the lowest level of normal. I diagnosed abdominal migraine and treated her thoracic spine. After eight visits she has remained free from attacks for ten years.

Patients like Mary who suffer from abdominal migraine and other diseases associated with the malfunction of the splanchnic ganglion are often amazed at their rapid recovery after treatment to the affected area in the back, namely the lower neck and upper half of the thoracic spine. Not only is there a marked improvement in their symptoms but they also feel altogether more energetic and better generally. They also lose the feeling of anxiety and tension which is often present.

It is very common for people with back trouble in this area to suffer depressions. This is because when the activity of the anxiety centre – stimulated to galvanize the adrenalin mechanism when it is suffering from a low output – goes beyond an acceptable level, the brain tries to resolve the problem with the sensation of depression.

As with all the ganglia in the body, which have various functions, one or more things may go wrong – mildly or seriously affecting a patient. This will depend on a number of factors, such as which part of the body is under greatest strain, which may have been injured, or infected, or subject to an inherited weakness. Most people do suffer to some extent or other. When I feel oedema around the splanchnic ganglion, I will ask the patient if he or she tires easily, has indigestion or suffers from dysmenorrhoea (heavy and painful periods). The answer is usually yes.

After treatment, the patients feel much more relaxed and freer in the physical area of the shoulder and spine. Indeed, as one patient said to me: 'I had not realized my back had caused so many other problems. I would put up with my painful back so long as I could continue feeling so much better generally.' Many others say the same kind of thing. Fortunately, the back pain is usually expunged as well.

Lumbar Sympathetic Ganglion

This group of nerve centres lie in the mid-upper lumbar region of the spine. Its functions are local, so there is no involvement of the patient's general health such as tiredness or anxiety when the nerve centres do not work as they should. The lumbar ganglion controls the flow of blood through the arteries of the lower part of the body and also controls the repair and maintenance in this part of the body. The two areas most affected by a breakdown are the hip and knee joints. For some curious reason painful knees seem to be a feature of people from ten to thirty, while older people tend to suffer more from pain and eventually arthritis in the hip joint.

ARTHRITIS OF THE HIP JOINT

'Please do something about my hip,' pleaded fifty-one-year-old Alice, who had been in considerable pain for two years. Her left hip was so uncomfortable she found it difficult going up and down stairs. She also had a problem lifting her left leg to get out of the bath and she suffered pain in her left knee after sitting for any length of time. The only way to relieve this was to flex the hip. Alice said she had tired easily for ten years or so and she felt depressed at times. Her blood pressure was high and it was being controlled by pills.

X-rays of the hip showed that it was almost normal. However, on examination, there was bad spasm in both her thoracic and lumbar spine. Alice had eight treatments on her back and hip at the end of which time her general health was much better. She stopped feeling depressed and her hip was no longer painful except occasionally after going down stairs. Her blood pressure required only about half the number of pills.

Why the diagnosis can be missed

Early arthritis in the hip joint can be very painful but, as with Alice, the diagnosis is often missed. This is usually for three good reasons:

- The first is that for some years the X-ray appearances of the hip joint can be normal. The original trouble is probably inflammation of the capsule (lining of the joint) and the soft tissues, which is followed later by wear of the cartilage of the joint surfaces. Normally, wear is repaired as it takes place. If there is back trouble present this wear is not fully restored each time, so there is cumulative wear.

  After, say, a year or so, some factor – such as sudden extra exercise or a jolt to the joint – alerts the ganglion to the fact that it has allowed repair to fall very far behind so it presses the alarm button for an emergency repair. This is called an inflammatory reaction and is associated with pain, which can be severe. The inflammation often spreads beyond the original area and in the case of the hip can even spread as far as the two big nerves that pass close to the joint.

None of this shows in X-ray pictures, although excessive wear of the cartilage can be deduced by the lessening of the joint space. Deformity and increase in the bone tend not to come until much later in the disease. Of course, the time scale varies a great deal from one person to another.

X-rays only show changes such as the narrowing of the joint space where the cartilage is worn and a change of growth or disease of bones and, of course, fractures. The inflamed membrane lining the joint and cartilage which can cause considerable pain cannot be seen on X-ray for a surprising number of years.

- The second reason that early arthritis is often overlooked is that the distribution of pain can be misleading due to the fact that a great deal of the pain in the hip is caused by the inflammation of two big nerves – the sciatic (see figure 7.5) and the femoral – that run across the joint and cause a disproportionate amount of pain in the leg. The femoral nerve has much the same relationship to the joint as the sciatic nerve but it runs in front of the joint and goes down as far as the knee. This will be discussed at greater length in the next section. The pain in the buttock is sometimes a cramp in one of the gluteal (bottom) muscles and so again the pain is not from the actual hip joint.

When the sciatic and femoral nerves become inflamed, the impulses sent to the brain originate at the site of the hip joint, but the brain does not realize this. It thinks the pain comes from the sensors in the beginning of the nerve, which lie in the legs, so that this is where the patient thinks the pain is coming from.

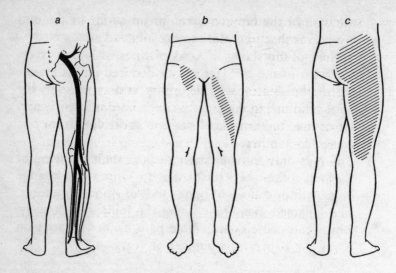

Figure 7.5 Inflammation of the large sciatic nerve is a common cause of hip pain. Diagram *a* indicates the sciatic nerve; diagram *b* shows the distribution of pain when hip arthritis is mild. Pain may also occur in the buttock; diagram *c* illustrates where hip pain can be experienced when the trouble is severe.

The usual nerve to become inflamed is the large sciatic nerve which runs across the back of the hip joint right down the leg to the toes (see figure 7.5). Referred pain from the hip tends to go down to the knees only although, if very severe, it can spread as far as the foot. Hip arthritis is a less common cause of sciatica than that which occurs when a nerve root is squeezed by a facet joint.

The other nerve is the femoral nerve that runs across the front of the hip joint down as far as the knee. This nerve becomes involved less frequently but, when it does, the pain may only be in the groin or radiate from the groin down to the inside of the knee. On careful questioning, the patient will often say that they have suffered from intermittent pain in the groin area alone for some years and that it is especially bad after exercising the hip joint.

● The third reason why the hip joint may not be suspected of being the cause of the pain down the leg is that the lumbar spine, being the underlying cause, is also likely to have been causing pain in the back. As we have seen, disabilities in the upper half of the back may be symptomless for some time but a problem in the lumbar spine makes itself felt earlier as this area of the back carries more weight and does more work. Thus, when a patient has had pain in the lumbar region for some years and then begins to have pain down the leg, the diagnosis of a prolapsed disc is tempting, although, in fact, the origin is in the hip.

To make this situation even more complicated it is far from uncommon to have two sources of referred pain, one from the back because a nerve root is squeezed in the neural canal, and the other from the inflamed hip. The inflammation of the nerve root in the back makes the rest of the nerve very much more sensitive – a light squeeze on the calf muscle can seem agonizingly painful. It follows then that what may have been a hardly noticeable problem in the hip joint can be magnified, causing the pain there to be unbearable.

When the patient knows best

Curiously, patients with arthritis of the hip often suspect that their problem may arise from the hip joint but their doctor may insist that it is a 'slipped' disc. It is, however, usually easy to distinguish between the two by the following analysis:

- **When the pain lies in the hip joint** the patient will often remember feeling an ache in the groin at infrequent intervals for maybe a year or so before the real trouble starts. Pain is felt in the buttock and down the leg to the knee. In severe cases pain can radiate down as far as the foot. It is also common to feel it in the front of the thigh radiating some way down from the groin towards the inner side of the knee.

  Hip pain is often improved by walking but may return after a certain distance as the walking irritates the joint. Sitting often produces pain. This is because the weight is taken by the joint and the sciatic nerve which is stretched across it, thus irritating the nerve. The pain may also limit the range of hip movements. It may especially affect the action of putting the leg out sideways and rotating the foot. Hip pain tends to come on gradually over many months and there are often intervals when no symptoms are felt at all.

- **Pain referred from the back** is often predominantly in the lower part of the leg, especially in the foot and calf (see figure 7.6). There may be numbness in the area. Hip movements are usually normal but patients may find it difficult to lift the leg with a straight knee. When lying on the back the leg should be able to go almost to a right angle. If the back is pinching the nerve root there will be agonizing pain down the back of the leg when it is lifted from ten degrees upwards. Standing, sitting and especially driving tend to aggravate the leg pain. Pain from the back usually comes on very rapidly, within hours or days.

  Both hip pain and the pain referred from your back are usually bad during the night and are often improved by exercise. The reason, of course, is that the poor

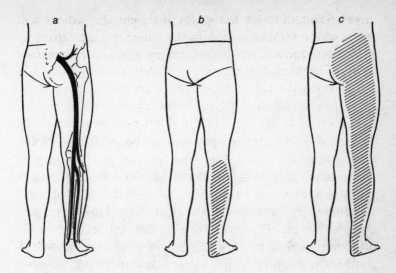

Figure 7.6 Various kinds of pain in the leg may have their basis in the back when pressure is applied to a nerve root. Diagram *a* shows the sciatic nerve, which is made up of many roots in the lower back; diagram *b* illustrates where referred pain is often felt when there is nerve root involvement; diagram *c* shows how the pain may be distributed in severe cases.

muscle pump during the night allows local pressures to increase. This interferes with the tissue circulation and starves the muscles of oxygen, leading to cramps. As soon as you get up and move around, the pressure is reduced and the pain improves.

How treatment helps

Treatment to the back results in the muscle in spasm returning to normal so that the muscle pump is restored. The lumbar ganglion therefore, being dried out, begins to work better at organizing the repair of the hip. Treatment to the joint itself, which is designed to improve the tissue circulation and lessen the spasm of the muscles across the joint, will, of course, speed up the effect of the treatment. For many patients, anti-inflammatory pills also reduce the number of visits required.

ARTHRITIS OF THE KNEE

The usual story of arthritis in the knee contrasts markedly with that of the hip. A young person will give his knee a slight twist doing some exercise such as playing tennis or squash or skiing. The knee may become painful and sometimes swollen but then clears up. However, the trouble then recurs with attacks of pain that become more and more frequent. Any trouble in a joint is arthritis ('arthros', meaning joint, and 'itis', meaning inflammation).

Local treatment to the knee may be enough to redress the balance in a number of cases. However, for the majority of patients, treatment of the back is also needed for more permanent relief. This treatment restores the ganglion to working order so it can effectively monitor repair of the joint. Of course, in some cases, the internal cartilage is damaged, but it is far more common that the cause of the problem is a failure of the repair mechanism due to the malfunction of the lumbar sympathetic ganglion. Another common cause is chronic tonsilitis. Bacteria living in damaged tonsils can put a toxin into the circulation which devitalizes any other membranes in the body which are similar to those in the throat. The membrane around a joint is particularly susceptible to this, especially if the joint is already slightly damaged.

James, a seventeen-year-old school student, was brought to see me with a swollen and painful left knee that caused him to limp. He thought that he had twisted it during a game of football some months before. It had been uncomfortable after the game and moderately painful the next day. His knee recovered after five days but two months later the pain returned for no obvious reason. The attacks became more frequent and severe until the last one, which had started ten days before.

His mother said that he had been having sore throats for many years but these had been much less frequent recently. The knee trouble, however, did coincide with the sore throats. On examination, his tonsils were large and unhealthy, although a culture only produced bacteria normal for the throat. I recommended that his tonsils should be removed. James agreed with my advice, his tonsils were removed, and I gave him some treatment with ultrasonic waves to the lymph nodes in his neck, which were enlarged and inflamed as a result of the long-standing tonsilitis. I was sure that the tonsils were the cause and, as with many other patients, removing them cured his problem. His knee problem slowly improved – with the help of some additional ultrasonic waves and exercise – until it was finally restored to normal after about three months.

It is very common for chronic tonsil infection to cause arthritic joints, a fact which often escapes the attention of diagnosing doctors.

ARTERIAL DISEASES IN THE LEGS

The lumbar sympathetic ganglion (the lowest of the sympathetic ganglia) controls the flow of blood through the arteries of the lower part of the body. A number of people suffering from lumbar pain complain of a sensation of cold or sometimes heat in the leg. There are, however, more serious diseases of the vascular system that are affected by the malfunction of this ganglion. One, where the artery is diseased and tends to go into a spasm during exercise, making any further movement painful, is called intermittent claudication. This is greatly aggravated by the excessive fluid in the region. Once the back has been treated and the underlying problem is relieved then there is usually a marked improvement in the distance the patient can walk without getting severe pain in the calf.

Can Anything Be Done To Help?

Although the symptoms I have described in this chapter are usual for these particular disorders, they may vary considerably and it is not practical to go into all the permutations in this book. However, I hope that enough information has been given for you to be able to distinguish the various diseases from one another.

The preceding chapters have given an account of many of the problems associated with a back that has been injured. Interesting as it may be to study the causes of these problems, the only thing that is of real concern to the patients is 'Can anything be done to help me, doctor?'

We now go into the final phase of this book to consider many of the various treatments available to back sufferers. Finally, I will provide a detailed description of the method that I have devised; although it may not always give *permanent* relief, it has helped almost every sufferer to return to a normal life.

8

BACK TO GOOD HEALTH

Treatment for your back problem

Physicians of the utmost fame
Were called at once but when they came
They answered, as they took their fees
'There is no cure for this disease'

By now you are probably becoming a bit impatient. I can almost hear you saying 'All this theory is well and good, but how can it be used to help my back troubles? Let's get on with it!' Indeed, I can fully sympathize with these sentiments. In my younger days, I had a bout of back trouble. It began as pins and needles in my leg and then I sporadically lost the use of the leg completely. At the same time I was suffering a lot of pain in my back. Like so many back sufferers, I was referred from one practitioner to another. Neurological, orthopaedic and physical medicine specialists all offered different diagnoses and suggested different treatments.

A Treatment that Works

After a year or two of unsuccessful treatment, I was getting most frustrated with the situation. 'Surely, someone must be able to help me,' was my constant plea. I duly did everything the various specialists told me to do. I even endured bed rest for a whole month. Osteopathy helped a great deal but each time the relief was only temporary. Traction made it worse. Nothing seemed to offer any effective help. Then, when surgery was recommended, I decided that enough was enough.

Having already spent some time treating patients with non-specific back pain I was convinced that the original cause of my problem was a fall down the stairs of a villa, during a holiday a few years before. So, I asked a GP friend to train with me for a few weeks and then asked him to work on my back using my directions. Within three months, I had made a full recovery.

Over the years, I have found that many patients who consult me have, like myself, already had several years of appointments and disappointments. 'I have tried everything and now I've been told that I must learn to live with the pain and inconvenience. Is there anything else?' is the common cry for help. In answer, this chapter describes a treatment which I have been developing for forty years, that offers reasonably permanent relief not only for back pain but also for the associated problems we have discussed on previous pages.

ANOTHER LOOK AT THE CAUSE OF BACK PROBLEMS

For a full appreciation of the treatment it is necessary to understand the cause of your non-specific back pain. I would like just to recap quickly on this before continuing. A past injury such as a fall from a swing or horse, a skiing or car accident, or a hard rugby tackle gave a jolt to your spine. The blow was largely absorbed by both an increase in the curve of your backbone and also by the elasticity of the discs. It was the stabilizing joints, the facet joints, which – because they were not capable of the same amount of movement as the discs – ultimately took the brunt of the blow and thus became bruised. As a result of the bruising, the muscles across the facet joints went into a powerful contraction called a spasm.

There is a mechanism in the body whereby impulses, originating in bruised joints, travel along the nerves to the spinal cord and then go straight to the muscles across the joint, putting them into a spasm. This produces an effect rather like a corset of muscles, which is designed to limit movement, thereby giving the joints a rest and speeding recovery. Unfortunately, in the case of the facet joints it is one of nature's bad misfires. In practice, the spasm puts enormous pressure on the facet joints and does very little to limit movement. The joints are not rested and every time they move, the strain is greatly increased.

This sorry state of affairs is greatly aggravated by the fact that an important function of muscles is of returning blood to the heart from the tissues. Every time a muscle contracts the tissues tighten both in the muscle and in adjacent areas. This forces fluid out of the tissue spaces into the veins where non-return valves ensure that it makes steady progress back to the heart. As the muscles in a spasm are permanently contracted, this pumping effect is interfered with and leads to excessive fluid, known as oedema, collecting in the area. The build-up of oedema has the effect of diminishing the circulation to the tissues, which not only delays recovery of the damage to the joints but results in even further deterioration. This affects tissues nearby, such as the sympathetic nerve ganglia, causing the related illnesses we discussed earlier.

Treating the Basic Problem

Clearly the basis of the problem is largely mechanical. The sufferer has bruised facet joints which have caused a powerful protective spasm of the muscles. Unfortunately, this keeps the problem going. It follows then that treatment must promote suitable conditions for the body to heal these damaged joints.

I believe this is most easily achieved at the present time by treatment with physical means like remobilization and manipulation, massage, cold, and ultrasonic waves. Physical medicine has the great advantage that, provided all reasonable precautions, such as X-rays, are taken, it has almost no risk and no side-effects. At this point, you may well be thinking, 'I've already tried those. They didn't work then so why should they now?' This is an understandable query often raised by my patients. In answer, I stress that it is necessary to distinguish between the tools of treatment and the treatment itself.

To illustrate this, consider Lego. Everybody has a number of different blocks. These could be regarded in the same way as instruments in physical medicine, such as one block represents massage, another manipulation, a third ultrasonic waves, and a fourth surged faradism. Now the generally accepted usage of these blocks might be to build a house – and this could be the normal use of physical medicine – but another person might make an aeroplane. The blocks are the same but the objective and the end result are quite different. So although the treatment involves the use of ultrasonic waves and manipulation, etc., the actual treatment is what is done with these. When employed by different people, completely different ways and results are achieved.

The Tools and the Treatment

The treatment of non-specific back pain is to make local conditions suitable for the body to be able to repair itself. The muscle spasm must be reduced so that some pressure is taken off the joints and the tissue circulation needs to be improved so that the stagnant oedema is squeezed out of the tissues spaces, making room for the fresh fluid to filter in. The ligaments also need to be stretched if relief is to be permanent. These tend to shorten, to take up the slack when the muscle is in spasm and the discs are compressed for a period of time. Unless they are made to revert to their former length they will continue to exert pressure on the joint surfaces and so interfere with treatment designed to take the pressure off the facet joints.

The 'blocks' that I have found best to achieve this are massage, remobilization, occasional manipulation, ultrasonic waves, surged faradism (this is best in the form of a square-wave pulse as the patient finds it more comfortable) and the application of cold.

NATURE'S CURE

If the facet joints are to be given the chance of recovery, the body's own emergency defence repair mechanism (discussed on pages 149–52) must be neutralized to a great extent. Nature's cure for a bruised joint is a protective muscle spasm and an inflammatory process. Before continuing, it is worth looking in detail at the functions and relationships of the various components of the normal circulation.

Consider the tissues as a town in the country, with the houses representing the tissue cells and the streets the tissue spaces. Cars, vans and lorries are the tissue fluids which carry fresh supplies, building materials and workers (i.e., oxygen, sugar and other essentials) into the town (the tissues) and take away the refuse (i.e. carbon dioxide and other waste products).

Now let us suppose that the town is only connected to the rest of the country by a railway line which, in the body, is the arteries and veins. When a train, which in this analogy is the blood, stops in the station (the capillaries), the train offloads the cars, vans and lorries from its wagons into the streets of the town. When they have performed their tasks they are reloaded on to the train, now full of waste materials, to be removed. And the process is repeated again and again.

An injury could be likened to a fire in a house in the town – the inflammatory reaction would be the attempt to deal with it. Messages go to the fire brigade and cause an over-zealous administration to direct a thousand or so fire engines to the blaze. These are accompanied by a large number of police cars, motorcycles and ambulances. At the same time it is business as usual for the normal population and traffic in the streets. As you can well imagine this may easily cause a traffic jam that could bring the whole system to a near standstill.

The number of trains increases and even extra lines to the station may be opened up but being unable to unload owing to the already crowded streets, the trains pass straight through the station. In the body, the excessive tissue fluid is such that it actually bulges the tissues, resulting in a local swelling. The inflamed tissues throb with the thunder of the extra blood supply.

People and supplies can no longer get through to the shops and the dustcarts can no longer collect the refuse. If the jam continues for too long, a partial breakdown in the ordinary running and maintenance of the town may well result.

This situation also happens in the body. Poor circulation

in the tissues not only delays recovery of the damage to the joints but also results in even further deterioration in them, also affecting tissues nearby such as the sympathetic nerve ganglia.

A wonderful new fire extinguisher would be of limited use to the fire brigade if it were unable to reach the fire. In the same way, an anti-inflammatory drug is often of limited value if it is unable to reach the tissue concerned. However, if a number of vehicles could be plucked from the streets by helicopters, there would be an immediate improvement in the movements of the cars. This is roughly what ultrasonics do to the tissue fluids.

Allowing for a bit of artistic licence, I will actually *squeeze* the town, reducing it to about two-thirds of its original size, and this will have the effect of shoving a large number of lorries and cars out of the streets back on to the trains to be carried away. This has an enormous effect on improving the movement of vehicles in the town and enabling the fire brigade to get through to the fire. In the body this is achieved by making the muscles in the area contract with an electrical impulse called square-wave pulse, or faradism, which activates the muscle pump (see pages 55–6). With the improved circulation, of course, the anti-inflammatory drugs can be a great help in speeding up the repair process.

OTHER TREATMENTS

Later in the chapter, I will discuss my recommended treatment at length (and if you wish to go directly to this, turn to page 203) but first let us consider some of the treatments available for people suffering from back pain:

- **Bed rest** is often recommended. A patient is put to bed and told to stay there until the pain has improved. However, as we have seen in previous chapters, this is not really a satisfactory long-term treatment. The lack of activity greatly impairs the circulation, which delays the recovery of the facet joints. Even if the immediate pain is eventually relieved after a period of bed rest, patients usually suffer from further attacks as nothing has been done to correct the basic problem.

- **Corsets** and in extreme cases, a plaster-cast, are a somewhat similar form of treatment to bed rest, as the main idea is to rest the back. If the pain is in the neck, a collar is used. There are certain occasions when this is the best form of treatment. They take a great deal of the load off the muscles, thus reducing their requirements of oxygen and food from the limited circulation that is available and offering temporary relief. One major benefit of wearing a corset or collar is the support it offers while standing or during a car journey; in general, they have the same disadvantages as bed rest.

A more drastic version of corsets are casts usually made of plaster of paris that act as a more complete support for the spine. They are heavy, hot to wear in warmer weather, and also make the wearer clumsy and partly immobile. They usually have to be worn for a few months, and then can be replaced by a corset. They can also be made of a setting resin which is stronger and lighter, but is more expensive and difficult to apply.

- **Traction** is also something of a double-edged sword. The advantages are that while the muscle is in traction the joints are freed from the pressure of the spasm and they have the opportunity to repair. However, the muscle pump often becomes even more inefficient while the muscles are in traction and so the joints do not always repair effectively. The muscles may also react badly to being stretched and go into a powerful and painful cramp once the traction is released. Some problems are helped by traction, others are made markedly worse.

- **Manipulation and mobilization** are used by various disciplines. Mobilization is a more gentle encouragement of movement of joints and tissues, whereas manipulation is a forceful thrust in the desired direction beyond the previously possible range of movement. Massage is the medical term for manipulation of the soft tissues and this can take many forms. Orthopaedic manipulation is a rather drastic way of trying to solve the problem. It is often given under anaesthetic and tends to be of a rather violent nature.

Physiotherapists. Many can mobilize or manipulate to a very high standard. I prefer the Maitland training, as it is very close to that which I do myself and is generally of a rather gentle nature (Maitland is an Australian who wrote a book regarded somewhat as the bible of physiotherapists). There are, however, medical schools who teach other methods.

Physiotherapists usually have equipment which they are skilled at using and that greatly helps in the treatment of back problems. They tend to employ physical means such as massage, hot wax, heat and cold, baths, shortwaves or microwaves, interferential electrical treatment, laser and exercises. They can usually get very good results treating back pain.

It is my belief that most people suffering from back and referred pain respond well to treatment with physical medicine, which has the great advantage of being virtually without risk. I have always had in mind the principle that 'the risk of giving a treatment should never exceed the risk of not giving a treatment'. As there is little or no risk to the patient from a non-specific back problem itself then little risk is justified in manoeuvres to relieve it.

Osteopathy. ('Osteo' means bone; 'pathy' means illness) was derived from bone-setting – a sort of intuitive manipulative treatment popular all over America in the last century, created by Andrew Still in 1874. He postulated that any interference with the nerve or blood supply to the tissues as a result of a structural problem such as a curvature or muscle spasm in the spine would prevent the normal 'self-healing' to take place. Treatment was to realign the structural and soft tissue problems that could cause the interference.

Chiropractic. ('Cheiro' means a hand; 'practos' means to use) is treatment by manual means. The treatment was developed – like osteopathy, from the American bone-setters – by D. D. Palmer in about 1895, and involves rectifying misalignments of the bones of the spine and other parts of the body to alleviate disturbances of the nervous system caused by them. Chiropractors do not use drugs.

Naturopathy. This treatment combines similar views to the osteopath concerning the relationship between skeletal realignment and disease, but it also concerns the belief that there is a need to help and reinforce the natural defences of the body by various other means that include fasting and diet, hydrotherapy, removal of physical tension to release psychological causes of illness, acupuncture, herbalism and homoeopathy.

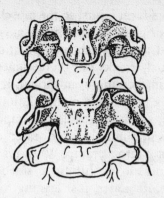

Figure 8.1 The strong, close-fitting and interlocking structure of the vertebrae makes displacement extremely difficult.

The manipulation is therefore similar or the same as osteopathy.

I believe that both osteopaths and chiropractors are giving the correct treatment for back problems, but possibly for the wrong reason. Both methods of manipulation have the basic aim of putting back displaced vertebrae. However, as figure 8.1 shows, the vertebrae are locked together most effectively. Indeed, it is hard to see how vertebrae can be displaced; if they are not displaced then there is no displacement to rectify.

Suitable manipulation by osteopaths and chiropractors does relieve back pain but this is not because it puts back a displaced vertebra. As we discussed in Chapter Three, the 'click' so often heard is, in fact, the freeing of a muscle which had become hooked around a bony projection. The moment the muscle is able to shorten, which is what occurs when my prescribed treatment is undertaken (see page 207), it starts to come out of cramp and the pain stops.

This kind of manipulation offers relief but it does not help the underlying problem. Nothing has been done to repair the bruised facet joints, so the muscles nearly always return to their original spasm and in most cases manipulation is needed again. Each manipulation will ease the pain of individual attacks but there comes a time when a muscle will go into cramp even though it is not stretched and it is at this point that manipulation can no longer relieve the pain, as the muscle is not trapped.

As conditions in a muscle deteriorate, it becomes easier and easier to put it into a cramp. When reasonably normal, something as drastic as lifting a sideboard would be needed to set it off. Later, just leaning forward could do it. When conditions are bad, it may go into cramp without being stretched – or the spine bent. It is then that it cannot be helped by attempting to shorten it, for it is already of normal length.

- **Drugs** used in the treatment of back trouble are mainly analgesics, anti-inflammatory drugs and muscle relaxants.

  Analgesics are simply pain-killers (pain-relievers). The most effective are the aspirin-like drugs, which are mild, but have the advantage of being anti-inflammatory as well. These have the disadvantage, however, that they can cause bleeding in the stomach and, very rarely, an allergic reaction.

  Paracetamol is similar to aspirin in strength but does not upset the stomach or have any anti-inflammatory effect. It is very safe, but can damage the liver if taken in excess. Liver patients should not take paracetamol.

  Co-proxamol (better known as distalgesic) is a much more powerful pain reliever, does not upset the stomach but has no anti-inflammatory effect.

  A much more powerful drug is dihydrocodeine (DF118). It can sometimes make the patient feel a little peculiar or nauseous. It is probably the most useful, however, when the pain is extremely severe.

Morphine, Phenazocine and Methadone are all very powerful pain-relievers but should be used with great caution – to relieve very acute pain as a means of tiding the patient over a short while until the attack is on the wane. The more powerful drugs can only be obtained by a prescription.

It is unfortunate that a very acute attack of pain is very difficult to alleviate with analgesics.

Anti-inflammatory drugs are a large group that work by preventing the production of the prostaglandins that stimulate the inflammatory reaction, which is the actual mechanism of repair. Unfortunately, it becomes so excessive that, as we explained on pages 183–4, it markedly interferes with recovery. Reducing inflammation therefore can actually help recovery to take place. There are a number of different substances which are in two main groups.

Steroids are very potent but are prone to cause side-effects if given over a prolonged period. Cortisone is the best known in this group. The NSAIDs (Non-Steroidal Anti-Inflammatory Drugs) are not so effective but on the whole much safer. Patients react differently to them so it is usually worth changing to another brand if the first ones tried either do not work very well or upset the patient. Many of them work vastly more efficiently if administered in the form of a suppository. All of them may cause indigestion or stomach bleeding as they inhibit the prostaglandins which confer a measure of protection on the stomach and bowel lining. Examples of these drugs are Brufen, Feldene, Froben, Indocid, Naprosyn, Ponstan and Voltarol; most require a prescription.

Cortisone injections are also somewhat of a mixed

blessing. They can be put directly – often combined with local analgesic – into tender trigger spots. They can also be injected directly into the facet joints or instilled around them, often by an epidural injection, so the injection goes into the space between the spinal cord complex and the bones of the spinal canal. This enables it to travel some distance without any risk to the spinal cord itself and to bathe the nerve roots and facet joints. The cortisone reduces the inflammation of the facet joints resulting in a reduction of the spasm. It is often administered for referred pain in a leg. If the patient makes a good recovery whilst the cortisone is active, he may well have prolonged relief of pain. Unfortunately, for some people these injections can cause deterioration of the joints, which leaves them in a considerably worse state. Subsequent injections seldom seem to help as much as the original one.

- **Injections of Sclerosing Agents.** This involves injecting a substance – such as a strong sugar solution that irritates the tissues, resulting in the production of fibrous tissue – which is designed to stiffen or stabilize the part of the back which is painful. These injections are really a form of built-in 'corset'. They are very effective in a number of patients but if they are not successful the patients may be even worse than before and the back problem can be more difficult to treat by other means.

- **Exercise** plays a valuable part in diminishing the symptoms of back trouble but as I pointed out in Chapter Four, I do seriously question whether it is of any help in actually correcting the basic problem. I see many patients who exercise regularly as instructed and still have their back pain. What is even more likely is that for a variety of reasons, perhaps a change of job or lifestyle, a patient will stop doing exercises after a number of years and the pain will return.

Aerobics are a form of exercise that involves many different pumping movements of the arms and legs. The recent development of Aquarobics and Aquacise (aqua-exercise) is much to be preferred as some of the unacceptable strain on the back is removed. Swimming is really a form of aquarobics as long as the strokes are varied a great deal. Disadvantages, such as having to hold the head up, thus putting a considerable strain on the neck, when employing the breast stroke, are thus minimized and the overall advantage of the weightless exercise is not counteracted.

See page 232 for some exercises to help keep fit and well.

- **Surgery** should, in my view, be restricted to those small minority of cases where there is a mechanical defect. This may be either a ruptured disc, two vertebrae that have slipped – one on the other – or a very unstable relationship between two vertebrae. The first needs removal, the other two stabilizing by means of a bone graft or screw.

- **Abraham's Box** (Radionics). The box is created around the belief that all substances put out a radiation and a human therefore puts out rays, which are made up of all the tissues in the body. If something goes wrong, the ray from the particular tissue is altered and this can be detected by the box. The box is then adjusted to give out a correcting ray, which will cure the patient.

- **Acupuncture** is a technique which originated in Ancient China and has been one of the mainstays of their medical practice until the present time. In recent years it has been widely adopted in Western cultures where it has many advocates. Some practitioners use the old Chinese theory of balancing rival forces in the body, whose imbalance has brought about a particular disease. This is done by implanting needles in a choice of sites on the body.

This has several medically understandable effects.

The first effect is that when the skin is punctured the body secretes a powerful analgesic called endorphines which tend to block the passage of pain impulses.

The second effect is that sensory impulses from the skin will block to a varying degree the passage of impulses up the pain-carrying nerves associated with this area. This is the same principle that you must have noticed when you have a painful spot and either press on it or rub it hard and the pain is greatly alleviated. This is also the basis of TENS, which we discuss on page 195.

The third effect is that if there is a great threat outside the body – such as a lion standing one hundred yards away – it is essential that the efficiency of the fight-or-flight mechanism is at its maximum, so internal pain such as an ache in the back or knee, will be inhibited (counteracted). Puncturing the skin could be the ultimate threat and so bring about a marked relief from the pain.

The fourth effect is that a barrage of impulses from a 'trigger point' sends impulses to the associated muscles causing a correcting redistribution of the chemicals in the fibres, resulting in the muscle relaxing from a cramp. This would, of course, relieve the pain of a cramp and by taking some of the pressure off the facet joint – if in the back – the conditions for this to repair would become much more favourable.

The fifth effect is that with some practitioners there may be an element of hypnotism brought about by the accompanying reassurance and constant suggestions that the condition may be improving.

Modern extensions of the simple insertions of the needles are also in widespread use – such as passing electric impulses through the needles called Electro-acupuncture – and these are said to enhance the effect. Acupuncture does seem to work for many people, although the benefits sometimes tend to be short-term.

Another variation of this principle is to heat the 'trigger spot' with a burning herb called Moxa. As soon as the glowing bundle of the herb feels hot it is removed. A smouldering Moxa stick may also be held near each 'trigger point' to achieve the same effect. The Moxa may also be burned on the top of the acupuncture needle so that the heat transmitted down the needle may enhance the effect.

A more modern variation of the acupuncture principle of pain-blocking by stimulating the skin is called TENS (Transcutaneous Electrical Nerve Stimulation). Small electrical pads are spaced over the trigger points and these are stimulated with a battery operated by a low frequency current. This can give considerable relief, even with severe pain, and has the advantage that it can be used by the patient at home or anywhere. This is very often used by women in childbirth.

- **Acupressure** or Shiatsu is direct pressure with a finger or knuckle on to acupuncture and other tender points. The effect is not as good as that obtained by using needles. A general massage is often given after the pressure treatment. This treatment has been derived from acupuncture in the last forty-five years. Originally it was used for relief of fatigue and as a general 'tone-up'. More recently, however, it has been employed both to diagnose and treat conditions similar to those treated by acupuncture.

- **Alexander Technique.** This was founded by an actor, Fredrick Alexander, about one hundred years ago in Austria. He found that his voice problems improved when he corrected a postural fault in as much as his chin projected forward more than normal. From this he developed a theory that from the original good posture and normal behaviour pattern of children we develop faults in the use of our bodies that interfere with the proper function of the muscles and nervous system. This results in poor co-ordination and balance. Common faults are tensing muscles, crossing the legs, jutting the chin forward and increasing the curves of the spine.

  Children originally are thought to imitate adults and thus acquire their bad faults. Treatment involves extensive retraining to correct the faults and it is the considerable commitment of time and effort that is the main drawback in an otherwise excellent and helpful system.

- **Aromatherapy.** This involves the use of essential oils derived from a variety of natural sources such as flowers, seeds, leaves, roots and barks. Several oils may be used in one treatment. The mixture of oils is concocted on a symptomatic basis, each being known to relieve its own particular complaint. The oils may be administered in several different ways – the most popular being combined with an overall massage or in the form of an inhalation. Many clinics, however, put the oils into a therapeutic hot bath. Recently a steam aromatherapy tube has been used, which is large enough to allow the patient to be completely immersed in the aromatic steam. The oils are very expensive because a great deal of work is needed to collect all the constituents and then to extract the essential oils. An oil like Neroli, for example, is drawn from orange blossom petals. Pounds of petals are required for only one ounce of oil. Fortunately, only very few drops are needed to make up the individual mixture for each patient. These oils are very potent and can be dangerous if taken internally. They should only be obtained from a reputable dealer.

Particular oils which are helpful for back trouble are lavender (in the form of a massage), marjoram and rosemary. Black pepper and ginger are helpful when there is acute pain.

- **Clinical Nutrition** (or Dietary Therapy). This has been considered at some length on pages 131–6. There is a belief that impurities in the system, mainly derived from processed and nutritionally empty foods cause arthritic conditions and back pain. This is dealt with by eliminating all these processed foods from the diet, often coupled with the administration of a 'cleansing' diet at the same time. Supplementary vitamins and trace elements are also commonly given to augment the diet. Some substances in particular, such as magnesium, calcium and potassium, may be recommended.

- **Healing.** This includes Faith, Spiritual and Natural

healers. Power is said to pass from the healer to the patient so that the patient's own mechanism heals the body. The source of power varies with the healer. Faith healers believe in using the patient's own religious beliefs to motivate healing. Other healers believe that they channel a 'divine force' or that they are directed by a spirit guide. Hostile influences such as anger are eliminated and the patient acquires a changed state of mind. There is no explanation as to what really happens but many cases of cures have been documented. Unfortunately, it is a discipline that is open to quackery so some caution is needed in the choice of a therapist.

- **Medical Herbalism.** This must be the oldest form of medical treatment, going back to Ancient China. Indeed, the medical pharmacopoeia is still largely derived from these natural sources. The main conflict between herbalists and doctors lies in the belief of the herbalist that the potency of the active ingredient is diminished both by purifying it and by the loss of the other substances in the herb which when present enhance its action. They also believe that synthetic copies of the original molecules are less effective.

  Doctors, on the other hand, are convinced that it is enormously preferable to have a substance whose exact effect is known and which, as it is pure, can be put into measured quantities ensuring that the patient receives a totally predictable dose. It has been found for instance that the amount of an active ingredient in a foxglove leaf (*Digitalis purpurea*) varies many times from one plant to another. A heart patient being treated by the leaf might receive either a serious overdose or one insufficient to help the condition.

Herbalists treat the whole body in correcting a complaint. Back pain is not really one of their strong points but the treatment may help. For instance, the application of silver birch bark may ease tender muscles, and a poultice of mustard seed relieves skeletal pain. An infusion of valerian will relieve pain, taken internally. Remember that some herbs may be dangerous. Only consult a registered herbalist.

- **Homoeopathy.** This therapy was started in Germany by Samuel Hahnemann toward the end of the sixteenth century. The orthodox treatment of the day was blood letting, drastic purges (having much the same effect as dysentery) and large doses of often toxic drugs. It has been estimated that the average mortality rate from the treatment alone was in excess of twenty per cent. This would have meant that if the patient had no treatment at all the chance of survival would have been that much greater.

  Hahnemann thought that taking substances that produced the symptoms of the disease, but given in very small quantities, would provoke the body's own repair mechanism. He postulated that medicines should not be mixed. Toward the end of his life he put forward the idea that the more diluted the solution of the medicine the greater the potency or effect. It is difficult to produce pain in the back with any medicine so homoeopathy is not an obvious choice for treatment, but several patients that I have been treating have been given an homoeopathic anti-inflammatory drug and this has proved most effective. There are also specific homoeopathic remedies for lumbago, coccydynia (pain around the coccyx), prolapsed discs, fibrositis, Paget's disease or ankylosing spondylitis.

- **Hydrotherapy** (Water Therapy). This goes back in the form of baths to the Greek and Roman days, as the heritage of baths all over Europe testifies. It can be beneficial both from the point of view of the exercise that can be undertaken in the weightless environment of the water, and also from various minerals in the water – either occurring naturally or subsequently added. In a number of spas the water is also drunk for its beneficial effect. There are many variations of the treatment as the water may be hot or cold – patients may alternate from one to the other. Jets can be used to stimulate the skin. Sitz baths employ the former technique and are very popular in health clinics.

- **Meditation.** Apart from any of the other benefits that this may provide, it does have a considerable effect by relaxing the muscles. It was shown that the tightness of the muscles has a considerable effect both on the likelihood of an attack of pain and also on the mechanism of repair. Meditation can be very helpful in both respects.

- **Reflexology.** The Egyptians amongst other ancient people believed that the body was divided into ten zones which were represented by different areas on the toes and fingers. This was further developed by an American masseuse, Eunice Ingham, in around 1930. She postulated reflex zones in a sort of map of the body and organs on the feet. A diagnosis could be made by ascertaining which of these areas were tender and treatment followed by administering deep massage to the areas involved. This treatment is said to be particularly helpful with neck, shoulder and back pain.

- **Yoga** is an Indian method of exercise designed to increase the life force in the body. It is an excellent system, which I strongly recommend to back sufferers. As in most exercise routines, there are a few movements that may stress the back and exacerbate the pain. These will become obvious fairly rapidly and can then be avoided. A Yoga teacher will be able to offer advice as to what is the best routine to follow. *Mantra* or *Nada* yoga is probably the best for pain-relief, as it affects the endocrine system.

AIDS TO MINIMIZE BACKSTRAIN

There are many forms of artificial aid to reduce strain on the back and you should consult a book specifically dealing with the subject for a complete list (see Further Reading, page 58). The following are, however, some of the most basic aids and forms of relief.

- **Shoes.** Special shoes can be helpful for correcting a variety of foot and leg problems. The shoe can be built up to correct a short leg; wedges can be put on a side to correct a tilt of the foot; bars can be placed across the foot to redistribute the weight better. The ensuing improved posture can help back pain a great deal. Cushions in the sole of the shoe can lessen the jolting effect of walking or running on manmade hard surfaces. This then eases the load on the facet joints and lessens the spasm during walking or jogging.

- **Seat lumbar supports.** In the majority of back sufferers, when sitting somewhat slumped, the muscles are stretched and this increases the tendency to go into a cramp. A support, pushing the lumbar spine straight, can go a long way to prevent this. Motoring is one of the most trying conditions for a back sufferer, so a lumbar support is even more beneficial in a car. People with stiff or painful necks can be helped, especially when driving but also sometimes when asleep. Prolonged sitting can make the neck very uncomfortable, so again a support may help.

Chairs are often designed more for appearance than for proper support. Really well-designed chairs are an enormous aid to comfort. Back shops are particularly qualified to advise on the best type of support for your particular problem. Choose chairs where you sit up with the lumbar region supported.

- **Beds.** We spend a large proportion of our lives in bed so it is worth spending as much money as you can reasonably afford on the bed. I recommend a good quality bed made by a reputable manufacturer. The most expensive mattresses are often so only because the coverings are costly and not because they are better in the spring department. A good salesman will be able to compare the supportive qualities of various ranges. Orthopaedic beds are usually too hard and, although better than a soft sagging mattress, may not give as restful a night as a firm grade of a standard make. The word orthopaedic has an interesting history. *Orthos* means straight and *paideia* means to train a child. The word derives from the time when many children had a tuberculous vertebrae. This would eventually collapse leaving the child with a horribly distorted – often hunchback – spine. A Welsh blacksmith called Thomas welded the children into an iron support that kept them straight for the year or so that was needed for the spine to heal. The child could then be released with a straight spine. Thomas's father became a doctor and as he continued to treat these children and straightened them, he was called an orthopaedic doctor – thus orthopaedics started.

- **Working surfaces.** Where possible these should be at a height that, when standing, bending forward is kept to a minimum. When sitting you should be able to sit up reasonably straight and keep the arms and hands at a comfortable height.

- **Loss of weight.** If you are ten, twenty, thirty kilos or more overweight, think of this as a normal-sized back sufferer going around all day with five, ten, twenty bags of sugar in a belt round his waist. Imagine the extra work your poor old back is having to cope with and without any increase of movement to keep the circulation going. It must have an effect on producing back pain even though it is almost certainly not the cause of the back trouble.

  A sensible weight-loss diet is the answer to relieving backstrain.

- **Massages and vibrating pads.** Wooden rollers with which to roll-massage the back can squeeze fluid out of the area and improve the basic condition. Vibrating pads and cushions also soothe the back and in moderation can do no harm.

A Logical Treatment

Now we come to the description of a treatment that has already helped many thousands of back sufferers. Admittedly, some patients are sceptical at first but afterwards they marvel at how the treatment has worked where all else failed. This is most rewarding, but I find it hard to share their excitement about the treatment. Given that the original cause is an old injury, then the treatment is so logical that its success is something to be expected.

SEEKING MEDICAL HELP

Before continuing I would like to stress that my treatment is for *non-specific* back pain. Also, that my work is done alongside, not instead of, other medical care. Back problems should always be given a proper assessment to eliminate all diagnosable causes. It is only after full investigations that a verdict of non-specific back pain can be reached. It is important that all back sufferers seek medical advice and help, especially over the complications that can occur with back trouble.

The various secondary effects of back trouble, such as a peptic ulcer or an arthritic joint, should also be medically supervised. These conditions may give rise to serious complications and it is important that the patient continues to be monitored by his own doctor or specialist during treatment to the back. The secondary illness will usually clear up within a few weeks of treatment to the back and nerve centres, but it makes sense to attack the problem on all fronts, especially if the local symptoms are bad.

HELPING THE BODY TO HEAL ITSELF

Every back problem is different, so it is obvious that no two patients can be treated in exactly the same way. The basic aim is, however, always to promote the repair of the facet joints. This depends on:

- reducing the muscle spasm as much as possible to take some of the pressure off the joints;
- improving the tissue circulation around the facet joints by squeezing out the stagnant oedema in the tissue spaces and allowing fresh fluid to filter in; and
- stretching the ligaments that have shortened during the muscle spasm.

The tools of the treatment are:

- **Surged faradism,** which has the effect of making the muscles contract and relax rhythmically at the optimum speed to activate the muscle pump and improve local circulation. Muscles contract and relax by stimulating the nerve which supplies them, in a graded increase and decrease. This may be the most important part of the treatment as the 'traffic jam' of fluid in the tissue spaces is the biggest single factor in delaying recovery.

Patients often comment that they can actually feel the muscular contraction and relaxation doing good, and although some feel slightly resentful that they have no control over it, the majority say that they know instinctively that this is exactly what their backs need.

Interferential treatment (a form of electrical treatment) that is often substituted by physiotherapists when asked to treat patients is not of any use for this purpose as it does not activate the muscle pump. The patients given interferential have almost all failed to make proper progress with their treatment.

It is important that faradism is not given at an uncomfortably strong level or carried out for too long –

the extra muscular activity would greatly increase the arterial blood supply. As the supply continues for some while after treatment has finished it would flood out the area again, impeding the tissue circulation and frustrating the whole beneficial effect of the treatment. About three minutes seems to be a good average time for faradism.

This story illustrates the need for moderation:

> The matron of my hospital, aged fifty-four, had broken her back a year previously. She was still in a great deal of pain so I was asked to see her. The fracture had healed completely but she was having severe pain in the muscles, which were in a protective spasm from the injury to the facet joints acquired at the same time as the fracture.
>
> I instructed the physio superintendent: three minutes of faradism, five minutes of massage, and ten minutes of ultrasonic and gentle remobilization to be given on alternate days. The next week everybody gave me black looks. 'I thought your treatment was supposed to make people better,' said a doctor. 'We are horrified; it has nearly killed Matron.'
>
> I sought the physio superintendent. 'What have you done to Matron?' I demanded. 'Well, I know you were trying to spare a busy department but as it was Matron I am happy to say that I was able to spare a physio every day. We also upped your almost non-existent treatment to something worthwhile – so we gave half an hour faradism, half an hour of massage and extensive remobilization.'
>
> It took Matron a fortnight to get over this so that treatment could be resumed. Happily, in the end, she made a good recovery.

- **Remobilization or manipulation** is another lynchpin of the treatment and serves more than one essential purpose.

1. Manipulation can relieve severe pain. The back is actually easier to treat when it is symptomless, but unfortunately patients tend to come to the doctor only when the pain has become unbearable. So before treating the basic condition, the pain must be eased. The most common pain in the back is due to a cramped muscle. Often this is aggravated by the fact that the muscle is hooked round a bone and remains stretched. This makes it even more painful and prevents it from coming out of the cramp. A suitable manipulation will free the muscle from the bone, often with a loud 'click', enabling it to shorten and quickly come out of the cramp.

2. Remobilization can free a nerve that is pinched in the neural canal. This occurs when the facet joint – which, as figure 4.2 on page 93 shows, forms part of the canal – swells into the canal and thus pinches the nerve. Mobilization or manipulation can open up the joint and so lift the pressure off the nerve and give almost instantaneous improvement in the pain.

3. Remobilization has a vital part to play in attempting to ensure reasonably permanent relief. When a muscle is in spasm the vertebrae are pulled together, thus compressing the elastic intervertebral discs. After a length of time, the ligaments contract to take up the slack. So, even when the muscle spasm is relaxed there is little improvement as the shortened ligaments continue to exert considerable pressure on the facet joints. Repeated, gentle, forced remobilization can stretch the ligaments back to the right length and help keep the muscle from going back into spasm.

- **Firm but gentle massage** both encourages the muscle to come out of spasm and squeezes the oedema out of the affected area into the veins, helping to normalize the circulation to some extent. The intensity of massage must be carefully calculated. It must be firm enough to produce the desired effects but not so vigorous or prolonged as to stimulate and increase the arterial supply (this will flood the area out later, as in the case of excessive faradism). Rub the back of your hand vigorously for a while and it will begin to go red. This is because of the increased arterial circulation. Well, this has the same effect as excessive massage deeper in the tissues.

- **Ultrasonic waves** are the most dispensable of the tools of treatment. These are sound waves that hit a far higher note than a human or even a dog can hear. Good ears can hear about 17,000 vibrations a second; the frequency I use is three million vibrations a second or three MHz, as it is expressed.

  When ultrasonic waves in a strength above about two watts to the square centimetre (a very weak dose) are applied to the muscles that are in spasm, they have the effect of contracting the arteriols somewhat, which lessens the excessive supply of blood to the area, and helps to get rid of the jam. On average, I use about five watts to the square centimetre, which is still a very small dose. In the early days we used to go up to one hundred watts, but this was often very uncomfortable and painful for the patient. The dose was gradually reduced until we reached the present level of below five watts – according to what and where it is being used; we found that therapeutically these small doses were just as effective.

  Ultrasonic waves also speed up chemical reactions,

probably by buffeting molecules about so they meet other ones more frequently. This, of course, makes the healing processes much faster. It is also thought to alter the filtration pressure of the tissue fluid by making some of the big protein molecules stick together, thereby increasing the pressure in the tissue fluid. This causes the fluid to be drawn out of the area, back into the blood vessels by a force known as osmosis.

Lastly, ultrasonic waves also encourage muscles to come out of a cramp or spasm. If they are applied directly over the facet joints, this greatly speeds up the repair processes. Patients find it soothing and most say they can actually feel the improvement. Patients will almost always improve without the use of ultrasonic waves, but the recovery will, of course, take somewhat longer.

- **A cold spray** or pack of frozen peas (petit pois are the best because they mould so well on the body contours) also helps, and this forms part of the treatment. The application of cold chills areas of the body and this closes down the arterial circulation locally (the body's natural reaction is to conserve heat by not allowing too much blood to become cooled).

This effect lasts quite a long time after the cold has been removed. As a result of this reduction in the arterial blood supply, less fluid enters the tissue spaces to replace the fluid that has diffused out. Therefore the tissue fluid pressure reduces and more fluid is able to flow through the tissue spaces. Repair is speeded up, so the cold has an actual curative effect.

Cold also reduces the sensitivity of the nerves –

remember the snake that could hardly move when cold? This means that the impulses that would have been transmitted to the muscles from the bruised area are greatly diminished and the protective spasm is therefore reduced proportionately. The reduction of pressure on the facet joints and possible slight improvement in the muscle pump also help speed up the recovery.

Of course, at the same time this major reduction in the conduction of the nerve impulses can greatly diminish the sensation of pain. This effect can be dramatic and by the time the nerves have recovered their function the other effects mentioned may well have produced sufficient improvement to have destroyed the pain altogether.

- **Anti-inflammatory drugs** may also be used in recommended doses if they offer a worthwhile reduction in the time required to obtain a good recovery. As we have already seen, anti-inflammatory drugs neutralize chemicals which produce the inflammation and can actually speed up the result of the treatment very considerably.

Answers to Some of Your Questions

How long does treatment take to work?

This is difficult to answer because, as the case histories in the book illustrate, there are considerable variations in the basic problem and thus the time it takes to regain a healthy back. Also, similar people with similar complaints can take widely different times to recover.

The total number of visits for treatment depends on

how fast the bruising of the facet joints recovers. This can be measured on palpation by the degree of spasm left in the muscles. When the muscle is completely free of spasm then it can be assumed the facet joints are fully repaired. It is unlikely that the original spasm will return again.

After the first treatment there is a marked improvement in the conditions needed for the repair of the facet joints: the muscles are more relaxed; they have refreshed fluid in them; and, the stale oedema has been pumped out of their tissue spaces. The joints will manage to heal a little and the spasm become less intense. Sadly, however, by the time they are ten to twenty per cent better, after only a matter of a day or so the body mechanism thinks it knows best and puts the muscles back into spasm, thus halting the repair. This necessitates another treatment to reactivate the repair mechanism. After each treatment the joints have the chance to repair more and more completely and so the spasm becomes less and less intense until it does not return at all.

Many patients are keen to know how I can be sure they are getting better. The only real answer is by palpation, to measure the amount of basic trouble still left. The pain may seem the same after several visits because the muscle may still go into cramp, but if the spasm feels as if it is lessening then I know that the basic condition has similarly improved. Treatment should continue until the spasm has almost completely gone.

As the joints improve, there is a corresponding reduction in the number of impulses travelling from the damaged areas to the muscles sending messages for them to contract; so, clearly the spasm is somewhat proportional to the level of trouble in the joints. The time taken for the treatment to bring about a full recovery varies greatly from patient to patient but most seem to average between six and twelve visits. Some need less, others many more sessions of treatment.

I've had back trouble for twenty years. Have I left it too late for treatment?

Patients with long-standing back problems are often troubled by the fact that it may no longer be possible for repair to take place. They feel that if only they had come earlier then something could have been done. However, given the right conditions, the body is just as capable of repairing the facet joints after fifteen or twenty years as it is after a month.

The bruising of the facet joints and the muscle spasm actually obtain a relatively stable state early on and this rarely alters much over the years. The spasm may very, very slowly cause the bruising to increase, but in general something of a status quo is established. As there is no built-in clock, the body is then unaware just how long the problem has been present.

Does it hurt?

The simple answer is no. In fact, for most patients it is very relaxing. For treatment to be successful it is important that it does not hurt. Pain is the ultimate alarm bell informing the body that something is wrong. Treatment must *not* stimulate this. If it does, the body will resist and eventually block the effect of it. Fortunately, very occasional sharp, momentary twinges, especially, for instance, the moment a muscle is freed, do not produce this effect.

How will I feel afterwards?

I have a rather black joke that in the early days of treatment the only certainty is uncertainty. Almost anything can happen in a mild way. However, the usual progress is that after the first treatment the patient feels a great deal better for a few hours and then the pain seems to come back, often just as bad as it was before. Despite this return of pain, the protective spasm – when felt by the practitioner – remains somewhat better and the patient is actually about ten per cent improved. After the next treatment, much the same happens except that the benefit may last a little longer. Again, the spasm is ten per cent or so less, which indicates a corresponding improvement in the facet joints.

The amount of pain that the patient suffers during the treatment can be affected by many things, including an anxiety state; participation in activities that can cause back pain, such as motoring; and even factors like food, drink and the weather. Patients may suddenly have a very good or bad day – neither is the actual measure of the real state of progress. The degree of spasm being generated by the inflammation in the joints is the only true indication of improvement.

After a couple of weeks, some patients may complain that they are getting no better. They say they are in much the same amount of pain as when they started the treatment. Indeed, they may still be in some pain, but often it is simply that having felt some improvement, they are now more sensitive to pain. As we discussed earlier, our pain threshold varies according to the circumstances. Remember, also, that your awareness in senses increases considerably after a rest from the stimulus. When you go into the fresh air from a room with a bad smell, or into the cold after time spent in a heated room, and then go back to it, it seems many times worse. In the same way, you can get so used to pain after a while that your body becomes less sensitive to it, but, given a period of improvement, then the same level of pain will seem considerably enhanced.

After a while, patients tend to have periods free of pain. Then, after a week or two they may suddenly have a bad day. The final twinges may not cease until two or three months after the last treatment as the large arterial circulation generated by the repair mechanism can still flood the muscles and cause a cramp. With the bruising recovered this circulation gradually returns to normal.

It is common for sufferers – especially those with upper-back problems – to feel very tired for some hours after treatment, or even the next day, following the first one or two treatments. After this, the opposite happens and they begin to feel better in themselves and have more energy.

Some patients, fortunately few in numbers, are made worse by the treatment for a short while. The treatment can feel slightly uncomfortable – massage, for example, involves rubbing cells together, and if these are badly injured they may not respond well. The overall effect of the treatment is vastly more beneficial than harmful but can produce a mild reaction, especially in the early stages before much improvement has taken place. This applies especially to migraine sufferers.

Others may feel no improvement for two weeks or so but, of course, the telltale lessening of spasm indicates the actual improvement and heralds relief from their symptoms.

My mother is eighty years old. Is she too old for treatment?

It is one of the saddest misconceptions that people become too old to have successful treatment. Indeed, the young and very strong are often the most difficult patients to treat. As we have seen, the main enemy of the painful back is the over-enthusiastic repair mechanism. If a person lives over the age of, say, sixty-five or seventy, they almost certainly have a good repair mechanism, to have survived so long. But, by now the adverse effects of a muscle spasm will have been greatly diminished with age and so will oppose the treatment far less. On the whole, older people seem to respond more quickly to treatment than their younger counterparts.

Where can I get this treatment?

The technique and equipment are available from a large number of physiotherapists. It is simply a matter of re-adjusting the use of their 'tools' to this slightly different way of treating a patient. It follows, therefore, that your own doctor will almost certainly be able to recommend a good physiotherapist who will have the surged faradism and possibly the ultrasonic waves. He or she should also be versed in the Maitland (an Australian physiotherapist who has written a book, describing manipulative and remobilizing techniques) or similar technique of remobilization. As the following section shows, this is extremely close to that which I have devised for my patients. As many osteopaths and chiropractors also have the necessary skills of manipulation, and use the same equipment, they will be able to give the treatment equally efficiently. See the following chapter for the details with which you can supply your therapist.

9

A NOTE FOR YOUR THERAPIST

*Working together to relieve
your back problem*

The apparatus and techniques required are as follows:

- **Techniques**. The ability to remobilize the back and joints in a manner similar to the Maitland technique, osteopathy or chiropractic.
- **Apparatus**. Surged faradic machine (preferably as a square-wave pulse) ultrasonic wave generator – any frequency will do but I have found 3M.Hz pulse the most satisfactory.
- **Massage**. Firm, but not deep, as it must not provoke an hyperaemia.

There is no particular order in which to give the treatment but it may be preferable to use the machines first if the patient is in a great deal of pain as it soothes the tissues and often relaxes some of the muscle spasm. If, however, the patient is not in severe pain, then the electrical treatment tends to relax the patient after the mobilization/manipulation.

Surged Faradism

The surge needs to be set at a cycle of about five seconds. I use pads about twenty-five cm long and five cm wide, and these are placed on either side of the vertebrae to activate the groups of muscles involved. Two or more locations may be needed to cover the whole area of the involved muscle. The intensity should be turned up gradually until it verges on being uncomfortable and then eased back a fraction. It is very important that the treatment is completely pain-free and comfortable; if the strength is excessive it will induce an hyperaemia which will continue after the treatment is over. As a result, instead of the tissue fluids being reduced so that there is a better tissue fluid exchange, the extra circulation will flood the area, defeating the object of the treatment. I have found that three minutes at each location is long enough to serve the required purpose. *Extremely* rarely this may provoke a reaction.

Ultrasonic Waves – Pulsed

This is given for a reasonable period of time at the discretion of the operator. Ten minutes over a moderately sized area (half the back or one hip joint) seems a good average. I use from two to five watts per square centimetre (w/sq cm) as this tends to reduce the arteriole circulation and has a maximal effect on the cramp – spasm, inflamed joint, etc.

I also use it on any secondary site of inflammation such as the knee, hip or shoulder joint.

Mobilization and Manipulation

This is applied both to the back and, if suitable, to any secondarily involved area such as the knee or shoulder. The strength needs careful assessing by test moves and only then should it be employed at the discretion of the operator. At the origin of the pain or elsewhere, a Grade V manoeuvre (manipulation) is often required. I use most of the following manoeuvres on the back.

1. The left thumb is placed with the first joint just below the vertebral spine, comfortably cradling it. The right hand is placed over the left thumb with it fitting comfortably in the hypothenar grove. Press to take up any slack and then push down using the arm and shoulder to give a firm sharp downward and horizontal thrust. All vertebrae should be treated in the area of the muscle spasm at grades III to IV, but tender spines or the ones suspected of being at the centre of referred pain should receive up to grade V.

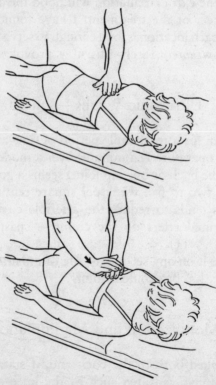

2. With pain in the low lumbar region, lift up the pelvis by putting the right hand under the ileac crest, and lift it about ten cm. Place the ball of the left thumb on the other side of the low lumbar vertebral

spines. Give a sharp thrust down with the left hand and a little up with the right.

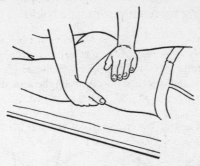

To do the other side: Stand on the other side of the patient and repeat the process.

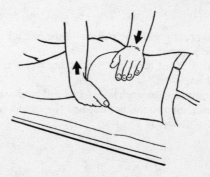

3. Place the patient on the opposite side to the known pain, the top leg in front and the top shoulder back. Pull the underarm as far forwards as is convenient. Place hand on the shoulder and the other

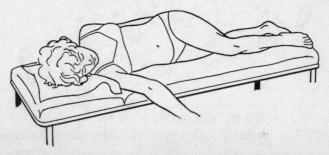

arm on the pelvic crest. Ease the patient as far as he/she can be rotated when relaxed. Take up the strain and give a moderate thrust in the same direction.

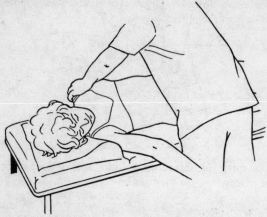

Repeat the other way with the patient on the painful side but this time use a grade V thrust.

Rarely the sharp thrust needs to be the other way – the patient feels the second one more.

If the pain is central – test each way – one will be more comfortable, the other often slightly increasing the pain. The comfortable side is the one to receive the grade V thrust.

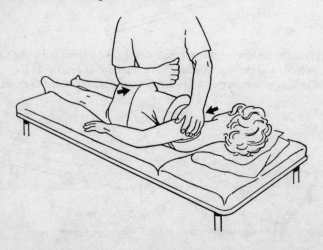

4. With the patient lying on his/her back and the couch head lifted somewhat, cup the chin with one hand and the occiput with the other. Make sure the teeth are closed and the tongue well clear and rotate the head in either direction. One way is almost always more comfortable than the other.

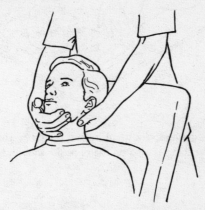

Rotate the head in the *less* comfortable direction using moderate traction at the same time. Take up slack – get the patient as relaxed as possible and breathing right out. Using the arms and shoulders give a thrust about grade III.

Repeat in the other direction, but this time grade V.

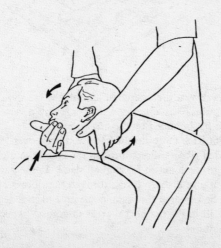

5. Place the patient on his back with the couch flat. The hand nearest

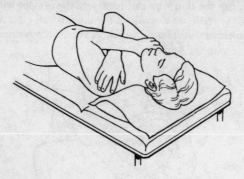

you is placed on the opposite shoulder and the other arm brought
over it so that the hand is also on the opposite shoulder.

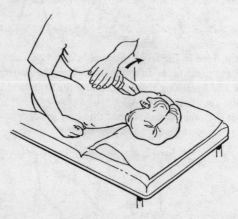

Stand roughly level with the mid chest and lift the far shoulder
with your outer arm. Place thumb on the back with a vertebral spine
between it and a fist bounded by the first finger.

Rest the patient back flat onto the hand and bend over leaning your
chest on the folded elbows. Press through the elbows and chest to
the vertebrae onto the hand to take up all slack. As the patient
breathes right out give a sharp thrust through the elbows and chest.

This needs to be repeated throughout the area of muscle spasm. I
vary from grade III in the peripheral areas to grade V where the back
or spines are painful.

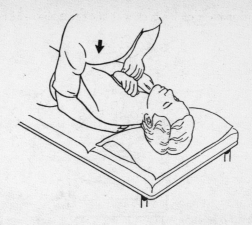

6. The patient sits on the couch with legs over one side. The buttocks should be well back on the couch. The patient grasps both hands behind the neck or if more comfortable places the hands just on the base of the neck.

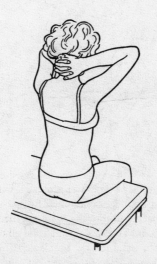

The operator threads his/her arms through the patient's arms and grasps the wrists firmly. The patient leans back on to the operator's chest and becomes as limp as possible. The operator thrusts the

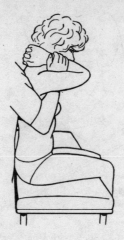

shoulders back and his/her chest forward at the same time, loosening the upper thoracic spine.

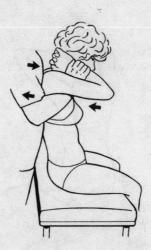

The same manoeuvre but this time taking up the slack in an upward direction. When the patient is completely relaxed the operator gives a sharp shrug of the shoulders lifting the patient sharply in an upwards direction.

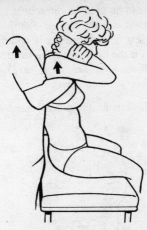

7. The patient sits on a stool with the operator standing behind. Place the left hand on the chin taking special care a) that the teeth are together and the tongue safely out of the way; b) that the inner part of the hand is not or will not press on the trachea which would cause the patient both discomfort and distress. Turn the head both ways – one is usually more comfortable. Start in the other direction.

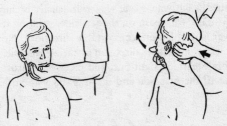

Turn the head as far as possible but using considerable traction at the same time. Give a thrust both round and up – grade III in the first direction and up to grade V in the other.

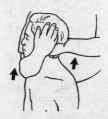

225

8. A variation of this can be used on infrequent occasions when a particularly strong patient is being treated. Put the right arm round the patient's chin cradling it (with great care and the same precautions as above). Rotate and lift the head steadying the occiput with the other hand. A sharp shrug of the shoulders gives increased thrust in the same manner as the previous manoeuvre.

9. Stand in front of the patient and place a hand on each shoulder.

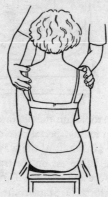

Rotate the patient each way – one way will usually be more comfortable (usually with pain on the left side, rotating the left shoulder forwards in the more comfortable direction). Now turn the patient in the less comfortable direction as far as possible. The patient relaxes, possibly breathing right out, and receives a thrust in the same direction grade III the first side and up to grade V the other side.

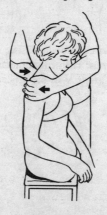

10. With very strong or unrelaxed patients, more leverage is possible by placing the near shoulder just past the chest, pressing the patient firmly towards one which locks that shoulder. Put *both* hands on the distal shoulder and repeat rotation as in step nine.

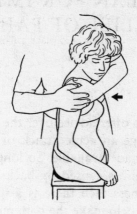

Indications for Manoeuvres

- Lumbar pain. Use the following steps: One (in the region of spasm of ten from sacrum to mid-thoracic), two, three, nine and rarely ten.

- Lumbar pain with tender thoracic spine as above, but also use five (especially on tender spines), and six.

- Neck and thoracic pain. Use one (in thoracic area), five (in thoracic area), six, seven and rarely eight.

- Neck and headaches. Use four, five (high thoracic), seven and rarely eight.

10

ACTION PLAN FOR IMMEDIATE RELIEF OF PAIN

I am often asked to offer advice over the telephone about how best to manage an acute attack of back pain until treatment can be made available. So long as your doctor is sure that the pain is caused by back trouble and not from any other illness then there is a number of things that you can do to help make the pain more endurable or actually to improve the underlying cause.

1. Try various positions for the maximum comfort. Often lying on cushions on a hard surface such as the floor can bring considerable relief.

2. Because muscles that are in a cramp do not like being stretched, a large cushion placed at the site of the pain will help. If you are lying on your side, the cushion under the more painful side is often best. Each case is different because the positioning that gives the most relief depends on which groups of muscles are actually in a cramp.

3. Try to move about: even if only to stand up and lie down again. The back gradually seizes up if stationary, so an effort to move should be made every half hour or so. As the pain improves, more movement will become possible and so the speed of obtaining relief will increase.

4. When the level of pain permits, try doing the exercises

on pages 232–3. If the pain is in the lumbar region (lower back) the rotational exercise for the lumbar spine will be the best. If your pain is in the neck, then try exercise 3 (see page 233) for the neck.

As the condition improves, more of the exercises can be incorporated into your routine.

5. A hot bath can relax the muscles and give considerable relief. Be sure there is someone around to help if the pain is so bad that you cannot get out of the bath unaided.

6. *Note*: General heat all over the body often helps but if it is applied to the painful area alone, it results in an increased arterial circulation at that one place – which causes increased oedema and a worsening of the overall situation.

This is usually true even if – by driving in extra fluid, oxygen and supplies – there seems to be a lessening of the pain in the first instance.

7. The application of cold lessens the requirements of the tissues by slowing metabolism and eventually it improves the local tissue circulation.

The best method for applying cold is probably a pack of something frozen – perhaps small green peas. This should be applied directly to the painful area and left long enough to chill it well. It is important that it is not left on for too long as frostbite may result. A minute would be a very rough guide. Of course, ice is very good but is less easily moulded to the body shape and may not give such a good contact as something smaller like peas.

Another very effective means is a cold spray. This should be applied very close to the skin to make a layer of fluid, if possible. This will also chill easily and without mess but has the two disadvantages of being expensive (the peas can be re-used) and the actual substance may be environmentally unfriendly.

8. Massage to the muscles may also be a great help in relaxing them and thus relieving the cramp. It is best done firmly but as far as possible without causing pain. The painful part of the back is often surprisingly unaffected by the immediate pressure of the massage.

9. Pain-killers, such as soluble aspirin, if this does not upset the stomach (it also has a useful anti-inflammatory effect), or Paracetamol, if the aspirin does, are good mild analgesics. Co-proxamal is stronger, but may require a doctor's prescription. The recommended maximum dose of these drugs must not be exceeded *however bad* the pain and the desire to alleviate it.

10. Most anti-inflammatory drugs need a doctor's prescription, although Nurofen can be bought from any good chemist and works well.

   The other anti-inflammatories are subject to the likes and dislikes of your own doctor. I use Voltarol (50mg), and find this drug useful. It is very much more effective as a suppository; in that form it almost never has any adverse affect on the stomach.

   All these NSAIDs (Non-Steroidal Anti-Inflammatory Drugs) have the disadvantage that they work locally in the painful area and, as has been explained on page 185, since the tissue circulation is poor as a result of the protective muscle spasm, they are often not fully effective until treatment has been commenced.

11. Muscle relaxants may also be very useful to lessen the spasm and thus also the cramp. They also tend not to work as well as theoretically possible because the cramp is a local reaction in the muscle and not influ-

enced greatly by the nerve supply. These are carbonate (Robaxin), and chloromezenome (Lobak), etc.

12. Finally drugs such as diazepan (Valium) have a powerful muscle-relaxing and general relaxing effect. They can be magic to abort a bad pain, especially in the neck or chest area of the back. They can, of course, only be given by your doctor – and for a very short while.

13. An injection of a local analgesic such as Marcaine (10ml), to relax the spasm can give immediate relief. This may well last long after the injection has worn off as the muscle is quite likely not to go back into a cramp. This will, of course, have to be administered by a doctor.

14. Lastly, there are two things which I often suggest that may give great relief to acute lumbar pain – providing the patient is an adult of normal or heavy build, is not fragile in any way (other than because of the pain), and has had back trouble on and off for several years. If there is a slight member of the family who weighs about five or six stone, he or she can walk with bare feet placed across the vertebrae up and down the lumbar and low thoracic vertebrae two or three times.

   The second option is to sit the sufferer on a medium-height stool, with his or her legs together (as in the diagram on page 226). A friend or family member stands in front with the knees between their legs (see diagram on page 226). Turn the shoulders each way; one will be much less comfortable than the other. Turn the shoulders as far as possible in the less painful direction and give a little push. This may well free the back with an almost immediate relief from the pain.

11

DAILY FIVE-MINUTE EXERCISE PLAN

Regular exercise increases the efficiency of the muscle pump, and keeps the muscles in good working order. A healthy body is a fit body, and chronic back pain can be kept at bay with gentle, daily exercise. Everyone needs and wants different amounts of exercise, so I will leave it to you to develop your own individual routine, incorporating as many forms of exercise as you (and preferably your GP) think proper.

The following is, therefore, the barest minimum of exercise which will help to keep the back – and only the back – in good working order. Anyone can do these exercises, whether or not you suffer from back problems. Even if you are able to move just a fraction of an inch, these exercises will help increase movement and flexibility, and reduce pain.

- **The neck**

    1. Turn the head looking from side to side as far as possible six times each way.

    2. Tilt the head from side to side as far as possible six times each way.

3. Rotate the head keeping the chin to the front six times each way.

- **The thoracic area**

  1. Rotate the shoulder girdle, with the arms hanging down, six times in each direction.

  2. Pull the shoulders backwards and forwards as far as possible six times.

  3. Arch the back pushing the shoulders back six times.

- **The lumbar spine**

  1. Rotate the lumbar spine six times with the arms out to the side at about forty-five degrees. At the extreme of each movement give the arms a flick in the same direction to give slight extra movement.

  2. Side to side. Lean over as far as possible first to one side and then to the other, six times.

  3. Arch the back as far as possible backwards, and then very slightly forward using the lumbar spine and hips as the pivot. Again do this six times each way.

12

YOUR BACK AND SEX

There was such an enthusiastic response to the first edition of The Back and Beyond *that we decided to run a telephone helpline to answer enquiries. One of the most revealing features of this helpline was that of the several thousand people who phoned in, around a third were having problems with their sex life: most commonly, pain on intercourse, tiredness, loss of libido and impotence.*

Until the publication of The Back and Beyond, *few of these callers had associated their sex life with their back problems. The book also prompted some of my patients to reveal that they had hitherto seen no reason to embarrass themselves by telling me about their poor sex life at the consultation. When they realised the connection they wanted to know more. This new chapter will shed more light on the subject by discussing the link between your back problems and your sex life.*

Back trouble does not affect the development and functioning of the sexual apparatus in either sex. The genitalia are controlled through their development and activity (i.e. producing sperm or ova/eggs by chemical messengers). These originate both in the Pituitary gland, which rests beneath the brain in the skull, and in the sex organs themselves; so they are all outside the effect of any back trouble.

The sex act, however, is a very different matter and can be affected in several ways by problems in the spine:

- Direct effect of pain
- Local effect of interruption of the nerve supply.
- Effects of Low Sympathetic Drive

These will be explained in full in this chapter.

Direct effect of pain

This is the most obvious connection. Anyone who has a painful back knows that certain positions are out of the question – even adopting the gentlest of poses can prove agony. Muscles don't like being stretched and sex involves a lot of bending and stretching. Some men complain that their backs are so painful they find it hard to keep going long enough to satisfy their partners, or indeed themselves.

> Jack, forty-five, came to see me with general backache. He said that one of his problems was that he found twisting and bending forward was most uncomfortable. He also mentioned that it was upsetting his sex life as he couldn't keep going very long – his wife was rarely satisfied and it had got to the stage where he wasn't reaching a climax either. He had tried taking painkillers but these had damped down his sexual sensitivity and made the situation even worse.
>
> The problem had started when he fell off a ladder a few years previously. Until then he had enjoyed a very good sex life and although his wife was very understanding, it was starting to cause tension between them.

Over the years I have come to realise that men are far less understanding of their partner's problems than women. Many women tell me that their backs are so painful they can take no active part in sex. Even lying still throughout intercourse is often unbearable. Yet, their male partners all too often fail to show any understanding.

> When Jane came to me she was suffering from lumbar trouble after a car accident in which she had been injured ten years before. She explained that one of the most unfortunate results of this was that she went through some considerable agony every time her husband, Gary, made love to her. The pain was severe when she moved in sympathy with him so she rapidly learned to lie quite passive during intercourse.
>
> Gary became very annoyed and upset and started to get critical. His attitude, together with the pain, made Jane less enthusiastic about sex. Gary began to have premature ejaculations and poor erections. In the end, Jane was completely turned off.
>
> Gary told her that he was working late more and more often until the day came when an emergency at home meant that she had to trace him. She found him in bed with another woman.

With correct treatment, Jane's back problem disappeared and her urge for sex returned. If only Gary had shown more sympathy and patience they could have continued to enjoy a happy marriage and fulfilling sex life together.

Local effect of interruption of nerve supply

The sex act involves a complex interlinking of nerves and minibrains which are situated at the lower end of the spinal cord. These are activated by both the brain itself and by sensory nerves that eminate from various erotic centres in the body. The most important of these by far are the cluster of nerves in the clitoris and parts of the vagina in women, and the tip of the penis in men. When stimulated, these nerve centres send impulses along the parasympathetic nerves to activate the sex organs. In the lumbar region the parasympathetic nerves pass through the spinal nerve canal along the second, third and fourth lumbar nerve roots.

If back trouble has caused the facet joints, or perhaps the intervertebral discs associated with these nerve roots, to become swollen, then this may have serious repercussions. The swollen joints or discs will press on the nerve roots as they pass out between the vertebrae and may well inflame the nerves at this spot. This can result in an interruption of the passage of the impulses along the parasympathetic fibres from the spine to the genitalia causing three main problems:

- **Lack of dilation of the blood vessels** which causes problems for both partners. An erection is brought about by impulses coming down from the back to the arteries causing a sudden rush of blood supply. This increased supply of fluid fills the space which is collapsed under normal circumstances and it expands over the entire length of the penis thus giving rise to an erection. When the nerve supply is interrupted the blood vessels do not dilate and men have a poor erection, or are not able to get one at all.

When women are affected by this problem they suffer from vaginal dryness and a diminishing of the vaso-motor effect on the clitoris and vagina. (Vaso-motor is the changing of the size of the blood vessels, by contraction or relaxation, of the wall of the artery). This is due to the same mechanism that causes an erection in men, i.e. an increased blood supply which fills the cavities to enlarge the clitoris and to expand a ring at the entrance of the vagina. Although this problem is not quite such a catastrophe as it is in men, it still makes sex less enjoyable for both partners.

Another effect of an upset in the control of the blood supply to the uterus is that it can lead to very **heavy periods**. However, it must be stressed that it is only when other causes have been eliminated that this should be considered. This increased blood also has another unfortunate effect. The liquid blood may clot because it has not been drained sufficiently rapidly from the very small tube of the uterus. These clots are removed, in the same way that a baby is expelled, by painful contractions.

- **Little sensation.** If the sensory nerves are interfered with in any way then this can cause the erotic sensations to be dulled for both men and women. This diminished sensation will result in men finding it hard to have an erection; even if they do then it is almost impossible to reach a climax. For women it is not such an obvious problem but the same applies and this lack of satisfaction may dampen any enthusiasm for sex. The big difference is that with the man it is obvious to both partners and this can cause psychological problems in as much as his fear of being shown up can in itself cause impotence.

- **Acute sensitivity** which makes sexual intercourse painful for both men and women. Acute sensitivity to light touch can give rise to pain in any part of the body if the nerve root is being compressed. In the normal course of events if someone touches you lightly then your nerve ending sends a few impulses per second to your brain which registers that you are being touched lightly. If you are being touched more firmly then the number of impulses per second increases to about fifteen or so. When you are being pinched the number rises to over twenty and your brain registers pain.

When the same nerve is being pinched half way along its length then the situation changes. The pinched nerve sends back a steady ten to fifteen impulses per second from the affected area to the brain. The brain largely suppresses this information as it is such a constant stream of impulses. However, if the nerve is touched and it sends back around ten impulses per second, these impulses combine with the steady ten to fifteen to make over twenty, which produces the sensation of pain.

In a situation where a person is suffering from compression of nerves in the back these nerves are already sending the brain a high quota of impulses so it only takes a small degree of sensation to turn touch into pain. This usually happens at the very last moment when the awareness of the sensation is maximal. Patients with back trouble complain of experiencing pain in the penis or vagina at exactly the wrong moment, making sex most uncomfortable. If this happens on several occasions then you will probably start to dread sex. For some men the extra sensitivity triggers off premature ejaculation.

Guy, thirty-two, has a lot of lumbar pain with some sciatica. On examination, he had a great deal of spasm of the muscles in the lumbar spine owing to considerable bruising of the facet joints. As he was nearing the end of his treatment, the spasm was very considerably less. About this time, he asked me whether my treatment could possibly have any effect on his sex life. When I asked him to explain he said that for several years he had been having a lot of problems and had been seeing a counsellor. He said that as soon as he went inside his wife he reached a climax. His wife was getting nothing out of their sex life. However, things had improved dramatically since the treatment to his back and his sex life was virtually back to normal again. This was, of course, because before treatment, the nerves in his lumbar spine were compressed thus causing increased sensitivity. Once the pressure on them was reduced, the sensitivity also eased.

PAINFUL PERIODS

This hyper-sensitivity can also be a cause of this distressing problem in females. The spasms of the muscles of the uterus often turn into mild cramps giving pain at the time of the period. In the same way that mild sensation can cause pain during sex, the discomfort or slight pain of the period becomes sharp pain for the sufferer.

Effects of Low Sympathetic Drive

As we have seen in Chapter 5, thoracic back trouble leads to a disease called Hypo Sympathetic Tone or HST for short. At this point you may like to read this section again to refresh your memory. One of the main symptoms of this disease is excessive tiredness which leads to depression. This extreme fatigue is hardly conducive to an enthusiastic sex life. It is no wonder that patients often tell me that they seek any excuse to get out of love-making with their partners.

Another symptom is a build up of excessive acid in the stomach which leads to problems with absorbing essential nutrients. One of the early casualties is Vitamin B. Lack of this vitamin adds to the problems of tiredness and inertia. It may also affect the ability of peripheral blood vessels to dilate – making it difficult to have an erection. It is the lack of dilation of blood vessels that also gives rise to the problem of cold hands and feet – and, far less commonly, to cold bottoms!

> Alice, thirty-six, had a problem with the whole of her back. She had aches between the shoulders and occasional attacks of lumbar problems with associated hip trouble. She said that the pain was having a profound effect on her sex life. It had got the point where she had almost given up.
>
> She also complained that she felt tired all the time and seemed to lack any inclination to make love. But the biggest problem of all, she confessed, was that she had an ice-cold bottom that boyfriends found most off-putting.
>
> Once her back was treated, all her problems melted away.

For Paula, twenty-three, the excessive acid in her stomach caused another problem – continual nibbling in an effort to mop up the acidity.

> Paula actually came to see me because she had a lot of aches between her shoulders. At the consultation she also revealed that she was eating all the time and was over three stone overweight. She explained that she felt so embarrassed to be seen in the nude that she avoided making love.
>
> When her back was treated, this hungry episode vanished. When I last saw her at her check-up she was losing weight and feeling much more self-confident.

HST can also cause amenorrhoea ('a' means without; menorrhoea means the monthly blood flow). This is probably brought about by several reasons:

- If you are feeling generally unwell then your periods tend to be scanty or dry up.
- The absorptional problems explained above can lead

to a deficiency in Vitamin B and Iron which causes the body to try to conserve blood by withdrawing the monthly blood loss.

- The imbalance between the sympathetic and parasympathetic can have the direct effect of limiting periods.

LOSS OF LIBIDO

The nerve complex in the base of the spine is influenced, apart from the sensory impulses from the genitalia, by tracts coming down from the brain. These have a very powerful effect on the output of the parasympathetic centres controlling the immediate sexual response. An erection can often be achieved, without the local stimulus from the genitalia, in a few seconds simply by the affect of thoughts, emotions, visual stimuli and odours.

Unfortunately this central affect can work both ways. Pain, whether in the back or the sexual organs, embarrassment or lack of confidence can have an inhibitory effect both on the desire to have sex and on the act itself. If the act of sex is unpleasant for whatever reason then the brain switches off the sexual urge as nature's way of finding an escape from a difficult or painful situation. This can eventually lead to impotence in men and frigidity in women.

Gladys, forty-two, came to see me because of back pain. She had fallen off a wall, flat onto her back, at the age of seventeen. Eight years later, she began to have low lumbar back pain. She had seen several practitioners but although she had been given immediate relief the pain kept recurring. Another problem, however, had gradually crept in and by the time she came to see me it had become a matter of the greatest concern. She had had pain so often when making love to her husband that she had begun to lose all interest.

She had no desire for sex at all. This was having such a bad affect on her husband that she told me her marriage was heading for the rocks. Fortunately things between them were not irretrievable and as her back recovered, her participation and enjoyment in love-making returned.

If you are feeling below par then the brain will also turn off your desire for sex. The law of the survival of the fittest means that anyone in a poor state of health isn't fit to have a baby. If you are feeling tired or depressed then you wouldn't want one anyway. So nature responds with a powerful turning-off effect for both men and women in an attempt to exclude conception. This has a greater influence in females than males. However, under these circumstances the male may well become impotent which is an altogether more dramatic result.

Clive, thirty-seven, had fallen off his motorbike nine years before he came to see me. He had some backache, mostly between the shoulders if he drove any distance or if he used his arms too vigorously. He tired very easily and had indigestion – he was being treated for this. He had also had two minor depressions during the last three years.

Clive needed eleven visits to get rid of the spasm in his back and alleviate all the other associated complaints. It was not until near the end of the treatment that he began to enjoy a most unexpected and positive effect on his sex life. For two or three years previously he had become progressively less interested in love making and more recently he had even been impotent on a few occasions. As he lost confidence, the problem got worse.

Now, for the last two or three weeks, there had been a remarkable change. His interest and desire had returned and he was having no more problems with getting an erection.

There is so much psychology involved with sex that if

you're feeling like sex but feel under pressure or simply want to please your partner then the whole episode could prove disastrous. And one failure can so often lead to another and a complete break down in confidence. Sex is an important part of a happy relationship. I have seen all too many people whose marriages have come apart because of the difficulties one partner finds in having sex. This must be one of the most compelling reasons for having effective treatment for a bad back, whether or not the back is painful.

This does not, of course, mean that treatment to the back holds the key to every sex problem. However, when all other possibilities have been investigated without success then a back problem should be considered.

GLOSSARY

Abdominal Migraine Episodic attacks of abdominal pain.

Abraham's Box A box which cures or controls illness by correcting faulty waves that the body produces while ill.

Acupressure Also called Shiatsu. Acupuncture points treated by finger pressure.

Acute Severe and sudden symptoms, with a quick resolution one way or the other.

Adrenalin Hormone that largely mimics the action of the sympathetic nerves.

Alexander Technique Treatment by retraining, to eliminate acquired postural faults.

Allergy Super-sensitive reaction to certain substances.

Analgesic Substance to eliminate pain.

Ankylosing Spondylitis Disease which causes both spine and hip joints to become stiff.

Anti-allergics Drugs to counteract allergies.

Anti-inflammatory Drugs given to counteract inflammation.

Antibody Substance produced by the body in response to antigens, which usually take the form of bacteria or viruses.

Aorta Large artery leading from the heart.

Aromatherapy Complementary therapy using essential oils.

Arteriole Very small artery.

Artery Vessel that takes blood from the heart to the body.

Arthritis Inflammation of a joint. There are many different causes.

Candida Yeast that infests the body causing problems like thrush.

Capillary Minute vessel that joins arteries to veins and which transmits oxygen and food to the tissues, removing carbon dioxide and waste from them.

Carbon Dioxide Gas resulting from tissue activity; it is released when we exhale.

Carpal Tunnel Syndrome Nerve pinched in wrist causing pain, numbness and loss of strength.

Cerebellum Little brain at the base of the skull that largely controls automatic repetitive actions.

Chiropractic Manipulating misaligned bones to restore health.

Chronic Disease lasting over a long period of time.

Chronic Fatigue Syndrome Also called ME (Myalgic Encephalomyelitis). An illness with many symptoms, the main one being tiredness.

Coccyx End bones of the spine forming the residual tail.

Congenital A condition with which you are born.

Cortisone Hormone secreted by the adrenal gland cortex.

Cramp Painful involuntary contraction of a muscle.

Depression The main symptoms of a medical depression are inertia, fatigue and sleeplessness.

Duodenum First twelve inches of the small intestine.

Electro-cardiogram An electrical tracing of the impulses from the heart muscles.

Elimination diet A diet which one by one eliminates various foods to discover a food intolerance.

Encephalon Brain.

Endorphine Chemical transmitters that influence (control) pain and other functions.

ESR test A blood test to check for the activity of certain diseases.

Facet joints For the purposes of this book they are the joints between one vertebral arch and another. The term applies to a number of other joints in the body.

Faradism An interrupted electrical current used to stimulate nerves.

Femoral nerve A large nerve running down the front of the thigh.

Fibrositis Non-joint rheumatic (or other) pain.

Flexion Bending a joint to approximate its parts.

Frozen shoulder A condition in which the shoulder joint becomes stiff and very painful.

Ganglion Virtually a small brain. There are many of these nerve centres scattered about the body.

Golfer's elbow A painful elbow due to a torn muscle insertion.

Hiatus Hernia The stomach bulges into the chest through an enlarged hole in the diaphragm.

Homoeopathy Treatment of disease by minute doses of substances which would produce the symptoms, and thus a cure.

HRT Hormone Replacement Therapy. Given to females after the menopause.

HST HypoSympathetic Tone. A new disease. See Chapter Five.

Humidity Increased water in the atmosphere, sometimes said to increase rheumatism.

Hydrotherapy Therapeutic treatment, including immersion and drinking, with water.

Intermittent claudication A disease of arteries in which they cut off the blood supply at times, usually causing pain in calf muscles.

Intervertebral discs Flexible, elastic pads separating the vertebrae from each other.

Ionization The forming of an electrical charge on an atom by adding or subtracting electrons.

Ligament Strong fibrous support connecting bones across joints.

Lumbar The lower part of the back, between the thoracic spine and the sacrum.

Lumbar curve The normal curve of the lumbar spine that gives it flexibility.

Lumbar Sympathetic Ganglia The nerve activity centres in the lumbar region.

Lumbosacral joint The joint between the spine and the sacrum.

Lymph ducts Tubes that carry the lymph from the tissue spaces to the lymph nodes and then back to the veins. The sewers of the body.

Lymph nodes The 'waste disposal' units in the lymphatic sewage system.

Magnesium A trace metal whose shortage in red blood cells causes tiredness.

Manipulation A sharp thrust to move a joint further than it previously could go.

Menopause The 'change of life' affecting women. The cessation of menstruation.

Migraine Very severe one-sided sick headaches.

Motor nerves Nerves which transmit impulses from the brain to the muscles.

Moxa A herb used to stimulate acupuncture trigger points, or to heat the end of an acupuncture needle, increasing its effect.

Muscle pump The squeezing effect of a contracting muscle to return the blood from the periphery of the body to the heart.

Myalgia Painful muscles.

ME (Myalgic Encephalomyelitis) Also called Chronic Fatigue Syndrome. An illness which causes, among other symptoms, great tiredness.

Naturopathy Treating illness with diet, exercise, hydrotherapy and osteopathy.

Nerve root Part of the nerve that goes from the spinal cord through the neural canal in the backbone to form a peripheral nerve.

Neural canal Space formed between vertebrae through which the nerves pass.

NSAIDs Non-Steroidal Anti-Inflammatory Drugs. Drugs that do not contain cortisone.

Oedema   Excessive fluid in the tissues, causing swelling.

Oesophagus   Eating tube which extends from the mouth to the stomach.

Oestrins   Female hormones.

Osmosis   Force that can draw fluid through a permeable membrane.

Osteopathy   Manipulative treatment of joints and soft tissues.

Osteoporosis   Thinning and weakening of the bones, mainly present in post-menopausal women.

Paget's Disease   A thickening of certain bones in the body, notably the skull.

Palpation   To examine the body with the fingers, relying on the sense of touch.

Parasympathetic   The nervous system that controls digestion, etc.

Pelvis   Several bones that have joined together to form a basin at the base of the abdomen.

Peptic ulcer   An ulcer of either the membrane lining the stomach or duodenum (intestine).

Physiology   The study of the workings of the body.

Physiotherapy   Treatment by physical means: massage, manipulation, electricity.

Platelets   Flat cells in the blood needed for clotting to take place.

Prostaglandin   Body chemical messenger. A wide range of effects, including increasing the inflammatory process.

Psychological   To do with the mind or mental activity.

Psychosomatic   A physical symptom caused or aggravated by psychological stress.

Pyloric sphincter   A circular band of muscle that controls the exit of food from the stomach.

Quiescent   Symptomless – the illness may be inactive or dormant.

Raynaud's Disease   Arterial disease causing an extreme reaction to cold, especially in the hands and feet.

Red cells   Cells which give the blood its colour and transport oxygen and carbon dioxide in the blood.

Referred pain Pain felt in a part of the body other than where it was produced.

Reflexology The diagnosis and treatment of the body weakness or illness by manipulating tender areas in the hands and feet, which affect particular body parts.

Sacrum Five of the lowest vertebrae joined to themselves and other bones to form the pelvic basin. The sacrum is part of the lower back.

Sciatica Shooting pain down the back of the leg, in the sciatic nerve.

Sciatic nerve Large sensory and motor nerve which runs down the back of the leg.

Sclerosing agent An agent producing hardening in the tissues.

Sensor Special organ at the beginning of a sensory nerve. Each one has a special function; for instance perceiving cold, heat, pain or vibration.

Serotonin One of the special messenger chemicals of the body.

Shiatsu Also called acupressure. Finger treatment of mainly acupuncture points.

Spasm An involuntary protective contraction of a muscle, but controlled through the nervous system and therefore symptomless.

Sphincter A ring of muscle to close a tube or orifice.

Spinal cord Huge nerve complex. An extension of the brain, passing down the neural canal formed by the vertebrae.

Splanchnic Ganglia Nerve centres influencing the viscera (bowel).

Spondylitis An active inflammatory process in the spinal joints.

Spondylolisthesis A condition in which one vertebra slips forward on to another.

Spondylosis A degenerative (wearing) condition of the vertebral joints.

Sterno-mastoid muscle Large muscle in the neck, from the base of the skull.

Steroids Chemicals related and with many similar actions to, and including cortisone.

Subconscious The very active part of the brain whose functions are unnoticed by the subject.

Surged faradism An interrupted electrical current with a rhythmical change of intensity. When applied to a nerve it produces alternating contractions and relaxation in the supplied muscle.

Sympathetic nerve chain An interconnected line of little brains that process the activity of the sympathetic nervous system.

Syndrome A group of symptoms and signs that constitute a definite disease.

Tendon The wire-like part of a muscle that joins it to a bone.

Tennis elbow Painful condition in the dominant elbow, caused by a torn muscle.

TENS Transcutaneous Electrical Nerve Stimulation. Using electrical impulses through small pads applied to the skin to relieve pain.

Thoracic To do with the chest.

Thoracic curve The curve in the thoracic spine that makes it flexible to absorb stress or a blow.

Thorax The part of the trunk between the neck and the abdomen.

Tissue fluid Fluid that has left the blood in the capillaries and is bathing the cells.

Tissue space The space between the tissue cells where the tissue fluid circulates.

Trachea The windpipe.

Traction Forceable pulling apart of the vertebrae (or other structures).

Ultrasonic waves A very high frequency sound wave, far above the hearing limits of the human ear.

Vagus nerve The main parasympathetic outlet.

Vein The blood vessels that carry blood from the capillaries to the heart.

Vertebrae Bones making up the backbone.

Virus Micro-organisms that can only survive in a host's living cell.

White cells Disease-fighting soldiers of the body. Found in the blood and lymphatic system, they are the basis for the immune system.

Yoga An Indian exercise routine to increase the life force, and flexibility.

FURTHER READING

Buchman, Dian Dincin, *Herbal Medicine* (Rider, 1979).

Chaitow, Leon, *Osteopathy* (Thorsons, 1982).

Davis, Patricia, *Aromatherapy: An A–Z* (C. W. Daniel, 1988).

Hendler, Sheldon Saul, MD, PhD, *The Doctor's Vitamin and Mineral Encyclopaedia* (Arrow, 1991).

Howitt-Wilson, M. B., *Introductory Guide to Chiropratic* (Thorsons, 1991).

Keith, Murnby, *Food Allergy Plan* (Unwin, 1985).

Keys, Sarah, *Back in Action* (Century, 1991).

Lockie, Dr Andrew, *The Family Guide to Homoeopathy* (Penquin, 1989).

MacKarness, R., *Not All in the Mind* (Pan, 1976).

MacKarness, R., *Chemical Victims* (Pan, 1980).

Mann, Dr. Felix, B., *Acupuncture* (Pan, 1973).

Newman-Turner, Roger, *Naturopathic Medicine* (Thorsons, 1984).

Nightingale, Michael, *The Healing Power of Acupuncture* (Javelin, 1986).

Norman, Laura, *The Reflexology Handbook* (Piatkus, 1988).

Olsen, Kristin, *The Encyclopaedia of Alternative Health Care* (Piatkus, 1989).

Royal Canadian Air Force, *Physical Fitness* (Penguin, 1970).

Stevens, Chris, *Alexander Technique* (Optima, 1987).

USEFUL ADDRESSES

London School of Aromatherapy
PO Box 780
London NW5 1DY

Back Pain Association
31–33 Park Road
Teddington
Middlesex

British Acupuncture Association
37 Peter Street
Manchester M2 5QD

British Chiropractors Association
120 Wigmore Street
London W1H 9FD

British College of Naturopathy and Osteopathy
6 Netherhall Gardens
London N3

The British Homoeopathic Association
27A Devonshire Street
London W1N 1RJ

British Migraine Society
178A High Road
Byfleet
Weybridge
Surrey KT14 7ED

British Rheumatism and Arthritis Association
6 Grosvenor Crescent
London SW1X 7ER

British Society for Nutritional Medicine
PO Box 3AP
London W1A 3AP

Nutri Centre
(Vitamins and Minerals)
7 Park Crescent
London W1N 3HE

Help the Aged
32 Dover Street
London W1A 2AP

International Institute of Reflexology
28 Hollyfield Avenue
London N11 3BY

Myalgic Encephalomyelitis (ME) Association
PO Box 8
Stanford-le-Hope
Essex SS17 8EX

National Ankylosing Spondylitis Society
6 Grosvenor Crescent
London SW1X 7ER

Institute for Complementary Medicine
21 Portland Place
London W1N 3AF

National Federation of Spiritual Healers
Old Manor Farm Studios
Church Street
Sunbury-on-Thames
Middlesex TW16 6RG

Research Council for Complementary and Alternative
Medicine
Suite One
19A Cavendish Square
London W1M 9AD

School of Herbal Medicine
148 Forest Road
Tunbridge Wells
Kent TN2 5EY

Society of Teachers of the Alexander Technique
20 London House
266 Fulham Road
London SW10 9EL

Yoga for Health Foundation
Ickwell Bury
Northill
Biggleswade
Bedfordshire SG18 9EF

19th April, 1990.

Dear Dr. Sherwood,

Having given my erstwhile wayward, and utterly unsympathetic autonomic ganglia a good airing recently in Texas I thought that I must write and thank you for what seems to me like a miracle cure. Whilst perhaps to you the treatment was routine, with no surprises, from my side of the ganglia it was a remarkable transformation, for which I am profoundly grateful.

Such now is my confidence in you that when I come to see you in June for a 60,000 mile service I shall expect you to press the right button to effect an instant cure for smoking. I feel sure that this must be within your repertoire.

With warmest regards and renewed thanks.

Yours sincerely,

PETER JACOB
Essex

INDEX